Conceiving Family

Conceiving Family

A Practical Theology of Surrogacy and Self

Danielle Tumminio Hansen

BAYLOR UNIVERSITY PRESS

Cover design and custom illustration by Hannah Feldmeier

Book design by Savanah N. Landerholm

The Library of Congress has cataloged this book under ISBN 978-1-4813-1056-7.

Printed in the United States of America on acid-free paper with a minimum of thirty percent post-consumer-waste recycled content.

To Eric,
the finest of partners

Contents

Acknowledgments

Many individuals participated in the process of conceiving, developing, and birthing this book. Carey Newman was an incisive, challenging, and motivating editor who empowered me to find this project's voice and helped me think about its content and structure in new and inspiring ways. My colleagues at Seminary of the Southwest offered encouragement and wisdom from their various areas of expertise—their doors were always open, their insights magnanimous. Shannon Craigo-Snell and Susan Brison read drafts of chapters and, along with Kristen Leslie, engaged in phone and email conversations to challenge and deepen the book's vision. Dale Andrews read chapters of this book on short notice and found time to meet in person to both affirm the book and also offer detailed critiques that strengthened its consistency and message. Candida Moss and Meghan Henning generously shared their own scholarly findings and encouraged this project to come to fruition. Natalie Wigg-Stevenson was an astute and generous conversation partner. Becky Watts was an intensely efficient and multitalented research assistant who eased the burden of writing and research in so many ways, and Greg Garrett offered fortification and reassurance.

I am also indebted to current and previous members of the Boston University School of Theology community. Shelly Rambo nurtured this project when it took a different form as a dissertation, as did Bryan Stone and Cameron Partridge. Claire Wolfteich, Kathe Darr, Marc

Lavallee, Stephanie Arel, and Alexis Felder all read the work at various stages and offered important feedback.

I give thanks for those who taught me about surrogacy and family through lived experience. Surrogates in the Austin, Texas, area generously shared their perspectives and indulged my abundant questions. While they are not referenced directly in this book, their openness allowed me to inhabit the surrogate world in a more embodied way, and it was a true privilege to gather with them. In addition, many adults who struggled with their own fertility shared stories that I did not discuss overtly in this book but that deepened my understanding of parenthood and the reproductive self. Finally, I am profoundly grateful to Marilyn, Bob, Marguerite, Gregory, Mike, Gail, Eric, Miranda, Andrew, Julie, Quinn, Elle, and Aidan, all of whom teach me on a daily basis what it means to be part of a family.

Introduction

Foundations for a Practical Theology of Surrogacy

The collective story of intended parents, surrogates, and children is one about dreams—dreams deferred and dreams realized. Humans thrive on their dreams, and sometimes their greatest fulfillment begins with the process of imagining what the future holds and who one will become in it. Some of those dreams evolve into unmaterialized fantasies, but others grip at the heart and become the basis for pivotal decisions that establish individual identity and solidify fate. That dream—the one that a person cannot abandon—may be an image of graduating from college or a vision of walking down the red carpet, or it may be the dream of something primal, something seemingly basic to the human condition: a life with a child.

A majority of those who dream of becoming parents have little trouble doing so, yet the dream seems beyond reach for others. The Centers for Disease Control estimates that infertility or reproductive loss prevents 12.3 percent of heterosexual couples from carrying a child to term, while same-sex or single individuals by necessity must utilize technology if they want a biological connection with offspring.[1] The quest to manifest the dream of parenthood is also frequently arduous for those who face biological obstacles: negative pregnancy tests, miscarriage, reproductive loss, the inability to imagine a future without children, and the sheer expense of assisted reproduction all tax one's body and mind. Meanwhile, the societal pressure to bear children presses against a fear that adoption is simply too complicated or may result in a biological parent requesting renewed custody of the child. Surrogacy is therefore often the culmination of years of unsuccessful pregnancy attempts, the last chance not only to become a biological parent but also to create a happy ending to the reproductive story for those who do not embrace adoption or childless living.

Surrogacy thus becomes the pen that individuals raise to complete a reproductive narrative that includes biological children, sometimes in spite of odds that imply biological children will not be possible because of reproductive difficulties, lack of a life partner, or involvement in a same-sex relationship. One might surmise, then, that surrogacy is rarely one's preferred ending to the reproductive story; rather, it is more often the last chance to reconstruct a story of loss as a story of gain, a story of conceded hope as one of hope restored. A theological examination of surrogacy is therefore partially an examination of how human beings use the resources available to them in order to write a narrative that transforms pain into joy. Yet it is also an examination of relationships and an examination of power because surrogacy necessitates relationships among intended parents, medical professionals, the woman carrying the developing human, and the resulting child that all wield it to different degrees. To complicate matters further, this subset of the reproductive economy is not produced in a vacuum: surrogacy practices represent the overarching beliefs and power structures of Americans.[2] How, then, ought one to think theologically about the dynamics of surrogacy to derive both focused implications for reproductive practices and conclusions that address society in a more expansive way? At stake in such a discussion is not simply the question of how one might evaluate reproductive technological power in the United States from a theological perspective but rather broader questions about the power dynamics in American society writ large. To that end, surrogacy may be said to function as a metaphor for the enactment of power in the United States. By saying something constructive about surrogacy, one can in turn say something constructive about American culture's use—and misuse—of power.

Method

To undertake such theological analysis is to embark upon a practical theological enterprise, for practical theology, as a discipline, aims to integrate practice with faith. Sometimes the practices under analysis are explicitly religious, and at other times they are not; sometimes Christian theology norms the practice, and at other times practice operates in the service of deepening theological claims.[3] Despite the discrepancies, many works in practical theology follow the same broad outline of beginning with analysis of the practice at hand, then turning to theological analysis, and finally culminating in revised practical recommendations. This book operates with the same general framework, beginning with a chapter that describes the contours of infertility, reproductive loss, the primacy of the biological family in the United States, and the reasons individuals choose surrogacy as opposed to other forms of reproduction of childless living, and then turning to a chapter on the construction of surrogacy.[4] The next two chapters provide theological analysis of surrogacy specifically through the lens of theological anthropology and collective sin; these chapters engage womanist and feminist thinkers to provide theological insights into what it means to be self in community, specifically communities with unequal power dynamics embedded in them. These chapters also rely upon the Bible as a source that Christians call upon for wisdom—using various tools of analysis for understanding that wisdom—as well as insights from secular thinkers in psychology whose wisdom offers a secular vocabulary for understanding what it means to be a self in community.[5] This wisdom from the social sciences is critically correlated with wisdom from the theological arts, with neither receiving normative priority over the other.[6] This project then culminates in a final chapter that synthesizes the findings from the theological reflection chapters to present an expanded vision of surrogacy that has implications for practices inside and beyond the reproductive sphere. Taken as a whole, then, this book moves from practice to theoretical analysis and then returns to practice.[7]

Limitations

Several limitations arise in such an investigation. Foremost, while this book discusses practices in other countries—especially India, which became a popular destination for assisted reproduction medical tourism, and Israel, which has a high rate of government-funded surrogacy—the focus is on the United States because it is the country with the highest annual usage of third-party reproduction and because it executes surrogacy in ways that make it distinct from other nations. These variations lead to culturally distinct surrogacy practices. For instance, domestic clinics usually demand a minimum payment for all third parties—be they surrogates or gamete donors—but intended parents may choose to pay substantially more in hopes of getting certain genetic characteristics in their offspring or achieving a successful pregnancy.[8] In no other country do either gamete donors or surrogates seem to receive as much as they do in the United States, with donors receiving, on average, a higher hourly compensation than surrogates. Intended parents in the United States also have more flexibility in terms of how they interact with and utilize the bodies of third parties: they can choose whether to keep third parties' involvement known or anonymous (a majority of gamete donors are anonymous), how many eggs to implant in a surrogate, and whether to selectively abort an embryo or fetus developing in the surrogate's body.[9] These prerogatives make it at least theoretically possible for a couple to hire an egg donor, sperm donor, and surrogate whom they never meet, to implant three embryos into the surrogate but decide to keep only two and require that the surrogate abort the third, and never to tell the resulting twins that they are not genetically related to the parents or that a surrogate carried them to term.

In contrast, other countries tend to have stricter regulations concerning third-party reproductive technology: Australia, the Netherlands, Switzerland, and the United Kingdom only permit intended parents to reimburse the expenses of gamete donors. Canada recently joined countries including Germany, the Netherlands, New Zealand, Sweden, Switzerland, Australia, and the United Kingdom in eliminating anonymous gamete donations, and a number of countries now impose limits on surrogacy as well.[10] China, the United Kingdom, Spain, and Canada permit altruistic surrogacy—surrogacy in which only expenses for the surrogate are paid—but deem illegal any kind of commercial procedure that results in the surrogate's financial gain. Italy, France, and Germany ban surrogacy entirely. India—a hotbed for surrogacy medical tourism—passed a ban on international commercial surrogacy, largely owing to ethical issues concerning the exploitation of women's bodies and unequal payment to surrogates abroad.[11]

In contrast to the aforementioned nations, the United States, federally at least, puts few limits on what intended parents can and cannot do when it comes to third-party reproduction. By and large, the desires of intended parents dictate their actions—finances allowing, of course—creating a free market for reproductive technologies that allows them to remain unfettered from the kinds of regulations that governments impose in other nations. Excepting individual states that have taken steps to regulate or ban surrogacy, the United States affords parents far more freedom than do most other countries with developed third-party reproductive practices.[12] The impact of that freedom to produce power and affect the types of relationships that develop—or do not develop—during surrogacy therefore becomes unique to the United States.

With that caveat, it would be remiss to forgo acknowledgment that this domestic context privileges intended parents with extensive financial means with the result that these adults are, in many ways, not representative of the demographics of the nation at large. The disparity between those who can access surrogacy and those who cannot emerges from soil that roots an enmeshed set of legal and social policies that privilege certain individuals. Insurance does not cover the cost of hiring a surrogate, which means that Americans who can afford a surrogate tend to be members of the upper middle or upper classes, and because of racial wealth inequality, they are often white. Most will have college degrees and some professional success; they are also likely to be older because they made investments in their careers before pursuing children, and by virtue of their age become more likely to have fertility problems, as reproductive difficulties spike in the late thirties, particularly for women. This is not to say that all individuals in the United States who hire a surrogate are white; it is not to say that all are over thirty-five or that all have a college degree. It is to say, however, that this is a common demographic among intended parents, so some of the claims made about American families in this work emerge from the priorities of this group. *Family* may mean something different in nonwhite America than it does in white America; it may mean something different in classes that cannot afford surrogates; and therefore the claims and issues that emerge from the definition held in those latter contexts may substantially differ from those described here.

In addition to geographic and demographic limitations, ethical issues related to abortion will be touched on tangentially. It may be argued in response that no research on surrogacy can entirely extricate itself from the abortion debate because it is impossible to escape the relationship between abortion and reproductive loss, given that both do not result in a neonate. Those who choose abortion take steps to terminate the embryo or fetus, while surrogacy procedures may result in the unintentional abortion of embryos or embryos that remain indefinitely frozen, never to culminate in a birthed life, though—given the fast-paced development of reproductive technology—it is not inconceivable that such by-products of the technology will be overcome. However, as that is not currently the case, the ethics of third-party reproduction and abortion can fluidly segue into one other—as the Vatican instructions *Donum vitae* and *Dignitas personae* observe—because both can result in embryos that do not culminate into a freely breathing newborn.[13]

There remain qualitative differences between the two events, however. The aborted fetus was to some degree unwanted, or at the very least, the desire for it could not counterbalance other concerns, be they medical, economic, or otherwise. The relationship between parent and aborted fetus is therefore a relationship from which the intended parent or parents explicitly sought to disengage or one to which they may never have consented in the first place.[14] In some cases, the process of aborting an embryo or fetus is an attempt by one parent or both to separate from the parental relationship with each other. It therefore functions as an act in which the involved adults—or teenagers—intentionally do not see relationships with each other as the conclusion to their reproductive story.

In contrast, the embryo or fetus involved in third-party reproduction—whether lost or not—may be considered the embodiment of relationship sought. Intended parents, doctors, surrogates, and donors all work together to ensure the creation of that life, and to varying extents in so doing, they create relationships with one another.[15] While there may be some overlap with issues surrounding abortion, then, explicit discussion of those issues exceeds the boundaries of this book.

Finally, many of the examples in this book draw from the use of surrogacy by heterosexual couples because of the book's emphasis on infertility and reproductive loss as motivators for it. Heterosexual couples are more likely to assume that they can procreate without the assistance of a third party, only turning to a third party when their bodies cannot reproduce via heterosexual intercourse. Surrogacy is thus often not the original plan for a heterosexual couple's procreation but rather becomes the plan when infertility and reproductive loss disrupt reproductive assumptions. These assumptions and the weight they carry figure prominently in what follows. In contrast, same-sex, transgender, and single individuals *may* not embark upon their reproductive journeys with the same assumptions and are perhaps more aware from the start that in order to start a family, reproductive assistance from a third party is needed, whether that third party be a donor, surrogate, or set of birth parents. The reason for using a surrogate and the surrogate's significance, therefore, may look different in the heterosexual couple's context because of certain assumptions about the reproductive process. It is therefore less the heterosexual couple qua heterosexual couple that this book aims to analyze than it is the meaning of personal fertility assumptions for family creation.

As the use of surrogacy becomes increasingly common, it is imperative to consider the theological implications of these procedures for the narratives of individuals, the construction of the self, and the families of which they are a part. Because if family is indeed the basic moral unit of society, then it stands to reason that how Americans define and exercise power in relation to the family may have extrapolative significance for other societal structures. In this way, the surrogacy system is important to analyze not just as a reproductive phenomenon but as a synecdoche for other American systems. A theological analysis of surrogacy, then, provides an opportunity for analysis of a certain manifestation of reproductive technology and also for some of our most pressing and haunting human needs.

As our world becomes increasingly strained by everything from wealth inequality to its growing population, the rising price of food and the decreased presence of farmland, violent conflicts abroad and within the home, strained race relations and unhealthy gender dynamics, theologians must consider again and again what it means to be a self, a self that exists in relationships influenced by cultural beliefs and practices that may clash with the fundamentals of Christianity. What follows seeks to become one small contribution to that timeless dialogue. It does so within two interlocking spheres, first by offering a new vision for relationships and power that can be employed by those who engage with surrogacy. Then, more expansively, it seeks to address those who wrestle broadly with the deep and abiding question of how to live in relationship with God and one another in contexts where power creates inequalities and where cultural misorientations instantiate entrapments that must be navigated in order to create meaning, freedom, and either literal or symbolic new life.

1

Infertility, Reproductive Loss, and the Significance of the Biological Family to the Self

Surrogacy is complicated for all involved parties—and perhaps that is why it remains relatively rare—yet some individuals still prefer it to adoption or childless living, raising the question of why. Why would a person go to such lengths to orchestrate reproduction? Arguing that reproduction is simply part of the self has its limits—given that some humans do not reproduce, and some have no desire to do so—and would require that one argue reproduction is an essential human characteristic or an essential component of the self, which might lead to the conclusion that those who choose to live without children are not fully human, or at the very least, that they lack a fundamental self component. Yet if an individual's desire for biological offspring is not rooted innately, then considering the impact of infertility and reproductive loss seems a worthwhile enterprise because it might reveal something about both what comprises the self and how these reproductive realities influence the decision to hire a surrogate. Such an investigation will also reveal how individuals process infertility and reproductive loss as it sheds light on how assumptions derived from the cultural construction of family affect that processing.

Reproduction and the Self

Contours of a theological discussion about surrogacy hinge on whether humans are essentially reproductive selves. Such a theological discussion therefore necessitates grounding in what characteristics are necessary for an individual to be considered a self, with the following discourse contending that humanness relies on the three characteristics of body, desire, and agency.

The Constituency of the Body

It may seem obvious to say that to have a self is to have a body, and yet complications arise when one tries to surmise what features that body requires. Genesis 1 might provide a theological starting point, for while it would be reductive to assume that the Bible absolutely grounds American cultural constructions of family, a plain reading of a text considered normative in the Christian tradition might still possess the potential to illuminate something truthful concerning the role of the body in relation to the self. Genesis 1 makes two statements of potential anthropological significance, the first being that humans are made in the image and likeness of God and thus should be able to form new life because God is prima facie a creator, having formed the world ex nihilo (Gen 1:27). Correspondingly, the next verse includes the first divine directive "to be fruitful and multiply," so that perhaps individuals who fail to do so lack a characteristic God intends humans to adopt (Gen 1:28).[1] If taken literally, these texts seem to imply that humans are essentially reproductive creatures with reproductive bodies, and so defined are they by that feature that it is one of the first claims made about them. Before the reader learns of the fall, before the human propensity for disobedience comes to prominence, before God identifies a chosen people or a savior appears in the narrative, what the reader knows is that humans are reproductive beings. Surely, therefore, the ability to reproduce must be an essential characteristic, essential to the body, for even if one puts aside these biblical accounts, reproduction is the very means of perpetuating the species. Humans can and have survived without ability to read; they can and have survived without the ability to farm, sew clothes, or fashion their own dwelling places. Without the ability to reproduce, however, the species would collapse.

By way of rebuttal, these texts can be read metaphorically. Perhaps one is meant to be fruitful and multiply in creative endeavors generally rather than reproduction specifically, or perhaps one is meant to share more expansively in image and likeness of God, rather than merely sharing God's ability to form new life.[2] However, even accounting for these readings, the inability to procreate is rarely, prima facie, of positive biblical value. Infertility is a source of suffering throughout both the Hebrew Bible and the New Testament: women such as Sarah, Hannah, and Elizabeth never celebrate their barrenness but rather lament it, and these texts describe children in terms of blessing when God steps in to provide them.[3] God never gives children as punishment but rather grants fertility and fecundity as rewards, the most paradigmatic example being that of Abraham, to whom God promises descendants numerous as stars and to whom God grants Isaac as a kind of ironic centenary birth present (Gen 18; 26:4). God even goes so far as to tell the people of Israel that those who remain loyal shall not experience infertility or miscarriage (Gen 26:4; Exod 23:26). To be unable to conceive or to be unable to carry children to term, then, seems to signal divine disapproval, an indication that a character is perfidious and deserves punishment. Children, in turn, become rewards. Yet such an argument can be made only if one accepts the premise that reproductive capability and children are both goods worth having. If one or both are of neutral or negative value, then it cannot be a source of punishment to deprive a person of them.[4]

The inability to reproduce raises questions about theological anthropology precisely because of such texts, introducing the possibility that someone whose body cannot create new life is somehow deficient because he or she does not possess the qualities needed to be fully alive.[5] However, biblical texts do not make the claim that the person who cannot reproduce is not human, even if one concedes that those texts suggest that fertility is a good worth having. Fertility may function as a reward, then, but this is different from saying it is an essential human characteristic: a teenager may receive a gold medal in ice skating, but this is not the same as saying that the essence of the teenager lies in her athletic ability. Rather, ice skating routines are acts that her body can perform in a particular way and with particular skill that might define her personality or her sense of purpose, but were she to break her knee and no longer be able to compete, she would not be somehow deficient as a human. Similarly, to evaluate humanness through a person's reproductive capability uses utility as a determinative measure. Christianity, however, has a long history of valuing human beings qua human beings—of privileging moralism over utilitarianism in this respect—and ultimately not valuing humans because of what their bodies can do or how well they can do it. To argue that humans are anthropologically deficient if their bodies cannot reproduce would therefore be to suggest that humans can be anthropologically evaluated on their ability to *do* something. Not only would such an argument call into question the humanity of prepubescent children and women who have undergone menopause—not to mention adults in their childbearing years who cannot procreate—but it would also raise the question of which bodily characteristics are necessary to inhabit the image and likeness of God and which are adiaphora. God speaks, for instance, repeatedly in the Bible; if a person is severely autistic, too young to speak or has a neurological deficiency that prevents speech, then is that person anthropologically deficient? And before taking the form of Jesus, God, as far as the Hebrew Bible documents, may have rested but did not sleep. Under such logic, every human who sleeps must likewise be considered lacking anthropologically.

One must also contend with Jesus who, as far as most Christian traditions believe, had a body that did not procreate. If God in the body of Jesus did not reproduce, then a compelling argument can and has been made that inhabiting the image and likeness of God does not require procreation either. To that end, theologians invoke this aspect of Jesus' life to explain the value of celibacy among monastics and priests. However, were one to question whether reproduction is anthropologically necessary, then celibate existence becomes theologically problematic because it would seem that God calls people to a ministry that diminishes them or somehow makes them less than fully human. Such a scenario in turn queries God's very goodness, for it would seem that God is simultaneously defining humanness by the ability to achieve a given end—reproduction—while issuing a call to celibacy that denies chosen individuals the possibility of inhabiting it.

Whether read with the plainest interpretation or read more expansively, scripturally based arguments for the fundamentality of reproduction for human identity fail to hold up because to argue that the body's inability to conceive or carry children to term is somehow determinative of one's status as a human being seems both counterintuitive and theologically problematic. It would require a utilitarian rather than moralist anthropology, wherein the ability to achieve an end rather than inborn dignity constitutes the main feature of humanness, and it would require that one delegitimize the value placed on celibacy in the person of Jesus and the various vocations within the Christian tradition that emerge from it.

While the body in general form is an essential characteristic of humanness, then, the reproductive capability of a given body is not, so that the presence of parts does not define the body but rather the integrity of the whole. And yet, the cries of Hannah to give her children or give her death alongside the other biblical accounts of barrenness illustrate the primacy of reproduction not just biblically but also in the lived experience of humans who yearn for children. How, then, does one explain the primal nature of this urge?

The Primacy of Root Desire and Its Translation to Projected Desire

The word *desire* often equates in casual discourse with *passion*, its connotation sexual. Yet the heart of desire, the root of desire, is not sex but self-preservation. Basic needs would go unmet if a person lacked this root desire—a given man would starve if he did not desire food or freeze if he did not desire clothes and shelter. A woman would burn her hand on the stove if she did not possess the desire to avoid pain, which is really to say if she did not possess the desire to continue living. Root desires therefore comprise yearning for the following basic needs, in no particular order: physiological needs, safety needs, social belonging needs (which include friendships, familial relationships, and romantic relationships), personal esteem needs, and self-actualization or self-transcendence needs.[6] Inherent in root desire's self-preservation is a level of self-protection and self-awareness that emerges from a sense that basic needs are not satisfied and should be. To that end, one does not necessarily desire what is good for loved ones or what is good for the species at large; the most primal essence of root desire is a desire for the self to survive.[7]

Only a casual observation of human experience is needed to recognize that people do not always desire what benefits their survival. Consider a stereotypical case of anorexia: anorexics present as desiring thinness, and the quest for thinness becomes so extreme that it can lead to health problems ranging from vitamin deficiency to kidney damage and fatal cardiac arrest. The desire for thinness ultimately becomes a vehicle that enables death rather than one that facilitates survival. Yet this desire for something other than life itself is arguably not the root of the anorexic's desire but rather the product of something that emerges from it. The anorexic may believe that she must be thin to be loved because of previous life experiences in which she was demeaned by others who did not perceive her to be thin enough, and to achieve their acceptance, she tries to meet their demands. The motivation for the anorexic's restrictive behaviors—not the behaviors themselves—therefore reveals the root desire of her actions, which here is the root desire to be loved. That root desire for love *is* generally beneficial to her survival (though perhaps she does not need the love of these particular individuals who insist on her thinness). The tenuousness of this situation arises when the root desire cannot be met, and the self tries to achieve it in a different way, projecting it into a form that could theoretically benefit her to some extent, even if it ultimately transmits to self-destruction. The projected desire—in this case, the desire to be thin—may bring about some benefit in the short term, but it ultimately does not act in the service of survival, nor is it what is truly sought. It is therefore a self-defensive measure but not a self-preserving one.

Projected desire may act in the supposed service of root desire, but it does not necessarily do so; it is both more malleable and more dangerous, and when one form of projected desire no longer serves or defends the self, it may be substituted for something else. For instance, a child in the foster system may have a wonderful high school music teacher who encourages her to sing in order to express the sadness she feels at being alienated from her family—in other words, to express her root desire for relationships. In this case, her desire to sing is a projected desire. However, when the foster teen gets transferred to a new school where music was cut for budget reasons, she may express projected desire differently, turning to opioids. The opioid high that initially seems to help alleviate her grief by letting her momentarily forget it can lead to overdose. This teen, however, does not overdose. Instead, she begins attending Narcotics Anonymous, at the urging of a school counselor, and stops using drugs, gets her grades up, and attends college.[8] In college, the girl majors in business because she wants to make sure she has skills that will help her get a job at graduation because she remembers the economic stresses her father experienced when he lost his job, which precipitated his abusive behaviors. Her projected desire for education therefore acts in the service of a root desire for physical security. That root desire for physical safety does help this young woman procure a job, at which she works long hours to get promotion after promotion, leading to an obsession with money and work—a form of projected desire—at the expense of relationships.

This example illustrates that projected desires may both benefit and harm the individual; they can provide short-term relief, but they often render opaque the root desire that actually needs to be satisfied. Projected desires therefore best achieve their ends when they express themselves in ways that are in the service of root desire as opposed to ways that sabotage it. How either projected or root desires becomes fulfilled, however, extends beyond the reach of desire itself and into the realm of agency.

From Desire to Agency

If desire signals the self's ability to be able to want for itself, then agency is the ability to pursue what one desires as a subject. Agency is both independent and relational so that the cognitive, emotional, and physical components of the self transfer into action. It is not necessary for agency to be successful for it to exist—a person can possess enough agency to act and still fail—rather, agency necessitates conditions that allow a person to take action in the first place. For instance, a sleeping baby may desire physical comfort, and a dirty diaper may be getting in the way. Agency, in this case, would look as follows: The baby would wake up and begin to cry. The mother might assume the baby is hungry and try to give him a bottle, and so the soiled diaper remains on the baby's body. Agency on the baby's part did not fail here, for the consequence of the baby's actions remains outside his control. That said, the baby will likely continue to exert agency—in this case, will continue to cry—until the mother figures out how to meet his root desire for a clean body.[9]

While the outcome of agency is not a necessary precondition for it to exist, the ability to act is, so that agential impingement occurs when one cannot act in the first place. A person taken prisoner may be tied to a chair to prevent escape, so that the person's desire for safety, a root desire, cannot be enacted. The captors thereby violate the prisoner by negatively affecting all three components (body, desire, and agency) of the self, for the act of restraining impinges on bodily integrity, is an affront to root desire, and prevents the exercise of agency to enact a root desire for physical safety.

That constraint placed on agency in this example changes the prisoner from subject into object. Yet a key component of agency is subjectivity.[10] As subject, the self as agent simultaneously requires independent movement and relational involvement, with the interplay between the two expressing themselves perichoretically. Both are necessary components of agency. As independent, the subject is capable of exerting agency of its own accord, unencumbered, with the ability to enact both salutary and damaging expressions of desire (the former being preferable to the latter). As relational, the subject chooses how and the degree to which other selves affect its expression. Positive relational influences help to construct the kinds of projected desires and agential forms that the subject expresses that not only benefit root desire but also that the subject welcomes. Friendship, in this regard, functions as an ideal form of relationality because it predicates itself on the mutual influence of subjectivity without a power differential between the parties involved.

Agency is essential to fullness of the self precisely because it establishes the person as a subject. As subject, the self can act, and acting is necessary in order to facilitate the root desires that are essential for survival. When something prevents the possibility of agency—whether wrought by natural forces or by another human—root desires cannot be sought, and if root desires cannot be sought, then survival cannot be achieved. Prohibiting agency, then, is an affront to the self's survival, an attempt to eradicate at least a component of it that can be either partially or fully successful.

The locus where agency and desire intersect becomes crucial to a conversation about infertility or reproductive loss. The body cannot satisfy desire in these scenarios because agency is unproductive. It cannot accomplish the task at hand. So even though the body can be considered a complete entity regardless of the ability to reproduce, if the desire to reproduce cannot be achieved through the exertion of one's agency, then suffering emerges because desire goes unmet owing to the subject's inability to act through heterosexual reproduction. Over millennia, individuals have tried to alleviate that suffering through a variety of creative alternative agential undertakings, ranging from at-home turkey baster inseminations to in vitro fertilization, gamete donation, and surrogacy. Understanding the history of surrogacy in turn becomes pivotal to understanding why humans turn to it when their previous agential attempts to meet the desire for children come to naught.

An Overview of Surrogacy

Surrogacy in Recent History

Approximately 12 percent of heterosexual married couples cannot become pregnant (infertility) or sustain a pregnancy (reproductive loss). Infertility tends to affect men and women equally, though the reason for infertility remains unknown in approximately 15–30 percent of cases.[11] Individuals must find different ways to create a family outside of heterosexual reproduction when infertility or reproductive loss prevents pregnancies from coming to term, with surrogacy being an option used over millennia. Most arrangements historically involved a husband physically impregnating a woman other than his wife to produce offspring that would be raised by the husband and wife as their own. This process allowed the husband to maintain a genetic connection to his offspring—and to produce legal heirs—while the wife achieved her status as a mother.

The economic and social contours of surrogacy in the United States began to shift in 1976, however, with the first legal agreement between a set of intended parents and their surrogate, all of whom remained anonymous from the public. This agreement outlined stipulations for the surrogate's participation in the pregnancy and the waiver of the surrogate's parental rights to the resulting child. It also stated that the surrogate would not be paid for her services. Formalized contracts such as this one eventually became standard in the surrogacy industry, codifying surrogacy as a type of formal business or legal contract. The changes in reproductive procedure, however, did not stop there. Two years later, Louise Brown became the first baby born using in vitro fertilization, and in 1983, the first ovum donation occurred. These technological advances foreshadowed an evolution in how Americans performed surrogacy itself, along with the contractual nature of its performance.

In 1985 a woman, whose name has never been published, approached doctors at Mount Sinai Medical Center about the possibility of combining two new technologies—egg donation and in vitro fertilization—to redefine surrogacy. The woman's uterus had ruptured twenty-eight weeks into a pregnancy, resulting in an emergency hysterectomy and the death of her premature baby girl from respiratory distress syndrome. Her ovaries, however, remained intact, and both she and her husband continued to yearn for genetic offspring, so they asked if it might be possible to implant an embryo fertilized with their ovum and sperm into the uterus of a friend who had previously birthed two healthy children. The resulting child became the first instance of a surrogacy arrangement in which the carrier's genetic material was not her own.

This new technology became known as gestational surrogacy, and it contrasted with historic forms of surrogacy—known as traditional surrogacy—that utilized the egg of the surrogate and the sperm of the intended father. Gestational surrogacy quickly gained traction with intended parents who simultaneously wanted to share genes with their offspring while also limiting the legal connection a surrogate might claim. Such procedures became even more popular following the well-publicized legal controversy of the Baby M. case, in which intended parents Elizabeth and William Stern hired Mary Beth Whitehead as a traditional surrogate. Whitehead claimed maternity rights following the birth of the baby, resulting in a highly publicized legal battle that eventually awarded custody to the Sterns while granting Whitehead visitation rights.

Gestational surrogacy remains the primary form of surrogacy in the United States today, and while heterosexual couples with reproductive difficulties often use it, it is an increasingly common choice for single individuals or same-sex couples who want to become parents. However, the legality of surrogacy varies by state, with some states permitting most surrogacy arrangements while others outlaw the technique entirely. As a result, those wanting to utilize a surrogate may have to cross state lines or travel internationally to do so.

Intended parents most often contract with a stranger to be their surrogate, though they also turn to friends or family members. Upon agreement, surrogates usually sign a contract agreeing to terminate rights to the resulting child and stating certain stipulations for the pregnancy, such as refraining from drugs and alcohol or being willing to engage in selective reduction or abortion if that is the will of the intended parents. In international arrangements—such as those in India—surrogates could be asked to undertake additional limitations, including living in a surrogate hostel and refraining from housework, heavy lifting, and sexual activity for the duration of the pregnancy. Intended parents, for their part, agree to cover all medical expenses for the surrogate and on average compensate them between $40,000 and $60,000, though the amount can vary widely. Previously successful surrogates generally receiving higher remuneration than first-time surrogates.[12] Surrogates are paid in installments, with some money distributed early in the pregnancy and the majority given after the live birth of the infant. It should be noted that when a surrogate is being used, she is not paid for her body.[13] Instead, she is being paid for the time and labor she contributes to the formation of the resulting child.

The Surrogacy Process

At the beginning of a gestational surrogacy cycle, both the egg donor—either the intended mother or a third party—and the surrogate begin to take birth control pills to synchronize their menstrual cycles. The ovum donor receives a single shot of gonadotropin-releasing hormone followed by daily shots of a follicle-stimulating hormone to increase ovum production.[14] Retrieval of the eggs takes place during an outpatient surgical procedure, approximately fifteen minutes in length, during which time the woman is fully sedated and a doctor inserts a needle through the vaginal wall and into the ovaries in order to retrieve the mature eggs. Meanwhile, the gestational surrogate takes daily shots of progesterone to stimulate the lining of the uterus for implantation.

At the time of ovum retrieval, the male—either a donor or the intended father—contributes sperm to fertilize the eggs. Medical professionals then fertilize a given egg with a single sperm, either by combining them in a petri dish or, if doctors are concerned about the quality of sperm, by selecting the healthiest ones and injecting them individually into the eggs. Three to five days after ovum retrieval, doctors implant the resulting embryos into the surrogate's uterus. The surrogate then continues to take hormones for several months until her body adjusts and is able to sustain the pregnancy on its own.

The surrogacy process is arduous, made painful by surgeries and daily shots. Yet surrogacy rates are on the rise despite the difficulties, outpacing the rate of growth for other reproductive technologies in the United States.[15] Perhaps the most obvious question that follows, then, is what compels someone to choose to participate in it in the first place, given not just the discomfort but also the cost. Adoption is often less expensive, and if one is concerned about the potential relationship with a surrogate, then one might be no less—or perhaps, no more—concerned about the relationships with adoptive parents. There are, at any given time, children already available for adoption through the foster care system, international agencies, and domestic agencies that help pregnant women find homes for their biological children. Yet surrogacy has become the preference for an increasing number of American adults in part because of the experiences that lead up to surrogacy and the effects of cultural views of the family.

What Is Reproductive Trauma?

Reproductive trauma is a phenomenon where negative reproductive events—including infertility and reproductive loss—lead to a trauma reaction in affected individuals. This is a relatively recent application of the term *trauma*. Social scientists used the word in prior decades to describe reactions to events that call the physical existence of survivors into question and which are accompanied by feelings of helplessness.[16] Instances of rape, violence inflicted during warfare, attempted murder, kidnapping, and other violent or life-threatening events are often described as traumatic, and indeed, in their aftermath, survivors may experience a cluster of symptoms that together constitute a post-traumatic stress response.[17] These may include flashbacks, intrusive dreams or thoughts about the event, a sense of foreshortened future, feelings of detachment or a desire to avoid trauma-related stimuli, and existential questions about safety and identity.

Given the kind of events that commonly elicit a post-traumatic stress reaction—events such as rape, warfare, genocide, and natural disasters—it may seem counterintuitive to reference trauma in relation to infertility or reproductive loss. Neither usually calls a person's physical existence into question—though some instances of reproductive loss, such as a ruptured ectopic pregnancy, might.[18] There may be neither the presence nor the threat of physical or psychological harm, and especially in cases of infertility, it is not the presence of something unwanted—an unwanted house intrusion, an unwanted sexual encounter, an unwanted bullet to the gut—but rather the absence of something desired that defines the trauma. Infertile individuals may be perfectly healthy and may not even know of their condition until they try to conceive, and indeed, if they had not wanted children, the condition might well cause less distress or potentially go unnoticed entirely.[19]

The second criterion of helplessness, however, is more clearly applicable. In cases of reproductive loss, women often feel powerless to stop a miscarriage or stillbirth as it occurs. They did not seek the pregnancy's termination—they desired this developing life—thereby differentiating reproductive loss from abortion. Women who experience reproductive loss specifically do not want the pregnancy to take this course, so the process of watching a developing life leave the body in the form of bloody tissue becomes a moment in which the body appears to violate the woman's agency. What was sought cannot be attained, what was desired cannot be achieved, and what was unwanted occurs despite best intentions. The processes of stillbirth and miscarriage thereby transform the woman's body from a site that creates life to a site that appears to destroy it, such that it becomes a liminal space, simultaneously living for her and a graveyard for the fetus.[20] Unable to make her body life sustaining, she finds herself powerless. Wanting her body to give life, she cannot intervene when it instantiates death, and incapable of altering the course of events, she is reduced to a bystander, a witness to the actions of her own body.[21] While such feelings may intimately touch women who were pregnant, their partners may experience helplessness as well, for reproductive loss also renders them onlookers who observe the departing of potential, the termination of the hope for children from the wombs of the women they love. These partners thus also experience a vulnerability wrought by desire that cannot transform to productive agency.

Helplessness also arises in cases of infertility, though it usually presents differently because pregnancy has not occurred. Approximately 15–30 percent of infertility diagnoses, for instance, have no etiology, no explanation for their existence, which can lead to feelings of disempowerment produced by the knowledge that doctors cannot explain what is preventing biological reproduction.[22] The ailment's origin is unclear, and therefore the reason for one's present suffering functions as a surd (something irrational or apparently senseless). This likens to the distinction between one doctor who says, "It's important that we cut your finger off, but I offer no further explanation," and another who says, "You have gangrene, and we need to cut your finger off." The diagnosis of gangrene provides a scaffold that supports a person's comprehension of why the limb needs to be amputated, much as knowing the scientific reason for infertility offers individuals a context through which to understand why they cannot procreate.

In addition to feeling helpless about how to contextualize the past or the origin story of the trauma, lack of an etiology also produces helplessness because there is less clarity about next steps. Returning to the analogy above, amputation makes sense when one knows that the limb in question has gangrene. There is not enough blood flowing to the area, perhaps, or dead tissue is now present, and long-term threats to mortality will arise if amputation does not occur. Understanding the cause of a condition may also allow the patient to be a stronger self-advocate, perhaps researching alternative, less drastic measures that could be used in gangrene's treatment, such as surgery to repair damaged blood vessels.

The same may be said for reproductive trauma. A woman who has a miscarriage because the child in question was not viable may be more likely to try again for a biological child, knowing the genetic issue that caused the miscarriage was rare and not likely to recur. A woman who experiences a miscarriage for no apparent reason has fewer resources that she can invoke in order to make decisions about her reproductive future. Similarly, a man who knows he cannot have children because chemotherapy from leukemia damaged his fertility may already have thought of alternatives to biological parenthood. In contrast, a man who has no idea why he cannot reproduce may have less immediate clarity on how to proceed.

The lack of known etiology may cause helplessness to transform into blame as individuals try to locate a reason for their suffering. It is therefore not uncommon for an individual facing infertility to attribute the condition to a past abortion, previous drug use or sexual partners, ambivalence about parenthood, or any number of other factors that may or may not have had anything to do with their present inability to biologically create children.[23] Some individuals may even reconstruct the meaning they previously formed of life events in order to make sense of infertility. Individuals may turn to "if only" thoughts to provide a context through which to understand the purpose of their experiences. "If only I went to the doctor earlier," or "if only I didn't go to the gym that day," or "if only I didn't eat so much sugar, since that's what causes infertility, even though the doctor said it doesn't"—such thoughts lay blame on the past in order to rationalize the present. They offer a cognitive mechanism through which a person might try to make sense of his or her own self-blame while seeking to provide an explanation for what appears to be an experiential surd. That explanation—however unrealistic it may be—in turn justifies what went wrong in the reproductive process. Infertility may cause a woman who was proud of delaying parenthood in order to establish a career and financial independence to become confident that her choice was self-interested rather than cautious. A man who believed it was moral to have sex before marriage and who participated in sexual activities with multiple partners may consequently wonder if his own inability to reproduce is a form of divine punishment because he did not stay celibate until he wore a wedding ring.[24]

Those who experience reproductive loss may also reconstruct their past to make sense of what otherwise seems ineffable. Unable to describe why a pregnancy ended, a woman may find it easier to blame a glass of wine consumed before she knew she was pregnant, or a man may blame an antidepressant taken years prior, instead of accepting that some losses defy reason.[25] Yet, as with other traumas, the instinct to blame is borne out of a desire to seek consolation through control, precisely because it provides a means to understand the incomprehensible. The trouble, however, is that the incomprehensible cannot always be explained, and that lack of explanation can, in turn, function as an irritant in the healing process.[26]

Existential Dynamics of Reproductive Trauma

Reproductive traumas can precipitate existential concerns, and while existential questioning is characteristic of trauma survivors, the types of queries related to reproductive trauma are distinct to some extent.[27] For instance, trauma survivors often find themselves questioning previously held assumptions about their safety in the world, and such searching makes sense in contexts where the trauma calls physical safety into question, as with sexual assault, attempted murder, or a physical attack. In each of these, the interpretation of the traumatic event arises in part because threats were made to one's physical safety, threats that violate commonly assumed norms of bodily security and autonomy. However, in many cases of reproductive trauma—absent those in which the mother's life may be at stake—bodily safety is not at issue. Still, such events can inaugurate questions about physical integrity that occur in response to the body's lack of reproductive success. The infertile man may have believed that he could reproduce until a doctor told him otherwise, while the woman who had a miscarriage may have assumed that she would be able to carry children to term. In the aftermath of such events, it becomes clear that these assumptions cannot hold, and as a result, individuals may feel as if the body has betrayed them and become unreliable.

In addition to questions about the body's integrity, previous successes in an individual's life may create cognitive dissonance with the body's current limitations. The typical infertility patient who seeks treatment at a reproductive technology clinic, for instance, often has a track record of being able to overcome hurdles and attain goals.[28] When reproduction becomes the goal, then, the inclination of such an individual may be to believe that it can be easily achieved, that it can be scheduled like any other meeting, mapped out like a vacation—sex on day fourteen of one's cycle means the baby will arrive in early May to avoid a hot summer pregnancy. Loss of control, however, emerges when procreation does not go as planned, when there is one stripe and not two on the pregnancy test and when the desire to avoid a swelling belly during the summer becomes, in retrospect, a frivolity.[29] The reality that one cannot control the body thereby grounds an existential clash between assumptions about what bodies should be able to do and what one's own body can actually do. This particular body should function the way all the others *seem* to do, the way that the woman's in the grocery store with one kid in the cart, one on a scooter, and one baby in a carrier apparently does. But the infertile body does not. The particular body's barrenness represents—literally embodies—a deviation from North American norms of what bodies ought to be. The particular body's limitations thereby make it difficult to maintain previously held beliefs about what the function of a given body may be.

Those who navigate reproductive trauma may struggle to understand the very purpose of their bodies in part because Americans are often raised with the assumption that humans are essentially reproductive creatures and that the culmination of one's adult sexual existence is procreation itself. What follows is a summary of the broad strokes of that cultural narrative: In procreation men, by nature, are able to offer sperm and women, by nature, are able to offer an egg and a womb.[30] Yet infertility and reproductive loss challenge such essentialist assumptions, triggering the cascading logic that a man may not be fully "man" if he is unable to produce sperm, and a woman may not be fully "woman" if she has no eggs or if her womb is inhospitable to the developing fetus.[31] The English language further reinforces the assumption that sexual or reproductive capabilities root one's bodily identity: if an individual breaks a bone, for instance, that person can say, "I broke my tibia," while someone who cannot conceive a child says, "I am infertile," not, "My reproductive organs do not work properly."[32] Language, therefore, explains the state of infertility as a problem related to the essence of being rather than as an action or an event involving an isolated organ within the body. In saying, "I am infertile," the individual linguistically adopts the status as a marker of selfhood so that it delineates reproduction as something intrinsic, rather than instrumental, to self-concept.[33]

Reproductive trauma also precipitates questions of ultimate meaning. Individuals may find themselves wondering about their own relationship with God and feel that God has let them down or that their diagnosis reflects God's disfavor. They may wonder whether they "tempted fate" by desiring children in the first place or believe that their inability to carry a successful pregnancy was a reflection of a kind of divine diagnosis of Unworthy Parent, as if God were using their experience of infertility or reproductive loss to send a message saying, "You are not good enough to raise a child." Individuals may question their previous choices, beliefs, and priorities or take stock of their existence in an attempt to measure whether it reaches a high enough mark for them to be worthy of parenthood by divine standards. Along the same lines, individuals may become concerned that their diagnosis occurred because their love as a couple was insufficient to deserve children, and that God used infertility or reproductive loss to prove the point. Hence, the sense of self one established over time is now not only being questioned but also being judged and, in being judged, found culpable. This may leave the individual or couple not only interrogating their identity but also wondering if the self they used to believe in was, in its very essence, good in the first place.[34]

The Narrative Self in Reproductive Trauma

Reproductive trauma affects identity in such a way that it may result in a crisis of selfhood. Janet Jaffe and Martha Diamond suggest that this crisis results from how one constructs a narrative of the self in relation to reproduction throughout the lifetime, a construction that they call the reproductive story.[35] Humans edit and revise the reproductive story throughout their existence, often rooting its first draft in their personal experience of being parented. Those with positive experiences of their mothers and fathers often imitate those behaviors, while those with negative experiences may define their future role antithetically to how their parents treated them. To that end, a man whose father always worked on the weekends may dream of being a parent whose schedule is flexible enough to allow him to spend time with his children more often, while a woman whose own mother was in an abusive relationship may commit herself to being a single parent in order to avoid an unhealthy dynamic with her spouse.

The narrative construction process begins in childhood, with children drafting their earliest reproductive story through play activities like putting a pillow under one's shirt to imitate pregnancy, protecting forts and castles from intruders, or having a "family" composed of stuffed animals, dolls, trucks, or trains. Play aids in the formation of a child's future parental identity and helps uphold the child's assumptions that he or she may grow up to become a parent.[36] Children thereby imagine adulthood from a young age. They mimic the actions of their parents and imitate their words or beliefs. They pretend to be doctors, astronauts, movie stars, and teachers. They play "house," and cast each other as the older sibling, the goofy baby, or the parent who swaddles dolls and feeds them fake milk from plastic bottles. These activities are not just innocent fun—they show the power of the imagination because it is through the imagination that children may test-drive potential adult selves and envision various futures in which they might participate.

After a time, children may favor one potential reality over another, resulting in particular choices that help manifest it: the little girl who loved to wear the toy stethoscope might take premed classes in college, while the boy who liked pretending to be a dad may start dating so he can start a family of his own. They then begin to test their reproductive identities—or their future parental selves—in more concrete ways as teenagers, through activities including dating, babysitting, taking on caregiving roles in the home, and, importantly, navigating sexuality and the possibility of parenting or the reality of it in cases of teen pregnancy.

Except in cases of teen pregnancy, common to both the childhood and the adolescent manifestation of the reproductive story is the way that it tends to image the parental self that one might become without yet realizing that self.[37] These stages of development may be said to function as a kind of prememory, or a future-looking image of what feels like an almost-inevitable reality that affects how one lives in the present. Prememory differs from memories of the past—which derive from recalled personal experience—and might more appropriately be related to the concept of postmemory.[38] Like postmemories, prememories do not derive from lived experience but rather are the result of inherited narratives or ways of being. However, while postmemories develop through the process of passing down—explicitly or implicitly—memories of the past across generations, prememory roots itself in inherited collective assumptions about what someday will occur. Prememories, like postmemories, affect an individual's way of being, causing a person to make specific choices or to adhere to certain beliefs, because of the power that these assumptions have.[39] Inherited cultural assumptions about the role of reproductivity in the life span may be said to function as such a prememory that affects the choices a child, teenager, and adult make, often to conform with the expectations that the assumptions set for them. In the United States, for instance, partnership and biological reproduction may be said to function as a prememory, as the assumed conclusion to a person's reproductive story—hence the countercultural status of celibacy. Thus, individuals often make choices about their education, career, and life partner with biological reproduction playing an implicit or explicit role. When some adults find that they cannot enact the prememory, then not only is their reproductive story without an ending but there is also a challenge to those prememories that shaped their decisions and, in turn, a challenge to fundamental assumptions about the sense of self that emerged from it. Many who cannot conceive or who experience reproductive loss did not expect such events; they were not written into the reproductive story they constructed for themselves in conversation with culturally derived prememories. Rather, they assumed the opposite, a narrative in which biological reproduction would be a given. The presence of prememories, therefore, affects the understanding of the significance of reproductive events including infertility and reproductive loss and may instantiate existential conflicts as a result.

The experience of such existential conflict is often confluent with the time when individuals seek a counselor to help them process the experience of reproductive events in their lives. Therapeutic best practices for reproductive trauma are nondirective, which means that instead of offering concrete advice or next steps, the counselor helps clients mourn what has been lost and then empowers them to write new endings to their reproductive stories that feel personally appropriate. In this way, individuals may develop an awareness of the prememories that they inherited and then make deliberate choices about the role they will play in their future reproductive narrative, given their body's inability to turn the prememory into a memory through biological reproduction. A new ending to the reproductive narrative must therefore be written that derives not from embedded prememories but from the discerned wishes of the individual. This new reproductive narrative may involve adoption, assisted reproduction, or childless living. These endings, like the earlier drafts, begin as dreams, able to be molded and shifted, but may also become realities.[40]

The therapeutic process is noteworthy in five regards. First, it acknowledges that what has been lost is worth mourning. The loss of a child one hoped to raise is worth mourning; the dream of getting pregnant is worth mourning. By acknowledging the loss, therapists validate the client's feelings and create space for grief.

Second, healing is not synonymous with the birth of a child within the therapeutic context; rather, healing occurs through the process of first mourning what has been lost because of infertility or reproductive loss and only then engaging in a process through which clients write new endings to their reproductive story that makes sense given the past. That story's ending does not necessarily require the birth of any child, let alone a biological child. It does not presume the inhabitation of the culturally dominant prememory, which presents the possibility that there can be multiple endings to the reproductive story beyond the one initially assumed.

Third, the process of rewriting the reproductive story helps clients see the ways that they still have a level of control over their reproductive future, thereby restoring agency in the aftermath of reproductive events that occurred despite intent and dreams. While individuals may have felt disempowered because they had no choice in how their bodies reacted to procreation, the therapeutic process provides them an opportunity to restore agency in a nondirective manner.

Fourth, the psychological process for treating reproductive trauma reflects those practices commonly used to treat other forms of trauma, thereby indicating that what humans process as traumatic may have broader dimensions than what was previously assumed. When treating post-traumatic stress in other contexts, therapists often employ a threefold system developed by Judith Herman wherein they first establish the client's safety, then help the client find ways to remember and mourn what has been lost, and finally encourage him or her to discover how to reconnect with the community in meaningful ways.[41] Reproductive traumas—unlike cases of domestic violence, say, or theft—may be less likely to require a therapist to help clients find ways to establish physical safety; however, they still benefit from engaging in the process of remembering, mourning, and reconnection that aids other trauma survivors.

Finally, the therapeutic process used to respond to reproductive trauma is significant not only in what it shares with other therapeutic processes but in what it does not share with medical ones. Here, a comparison between the way a therapist interacts with a client who experienced infertility or reproductive loss differs from that of a medical doctor: For the medical community, the solution to a given person's infertility or reproductive loss is to exhaust all possible scientific measures that allow a person to create biological offspring, and the manifestation of healing comes when that new biological life is birthed successfully in the manner desired by the potential parents.[42] This is the job of the infertility specialist or medical endocrinologist. In contrast, the therapist's vision of a successful conclusion following reproductive trauma is far less directive, open to the discernment of the client in such a way that might equally privilege biological parenthood, adoptive parenthood, or the decision not to have children at all. Such differences may result from pragmatics: the therapist's paycheck does not depend on the utilization of certain procedures, whereas the infertility doctor would suffer financial losses if the practice's clients decided to remain childless or adopt. However, it may be that the medical vision for healing is less mercenary than that. It may be that this perspective derives from widely held American assumptions about the family itself.

The Supremacy of the Biological Family Model

The United States has a long history of privileging biological family. Couples historically preferred biological offspring to adopted ones both because inheritance laws stated that estates could be passed only to blood relatives and because large families signaled prosperity.[43] While the value of biological inheritance still dominates in the United States, the value of large families has decreased. Beginning in the nineteenth century, advances in birth control and abortion technology led to a decline in family size, and more recently other factors—including the cost of raising a child, the possibility of women's work outside the home, an increase in childbearing age, and environmental concerns—also contributed. To that end the number of children per couple in the United States dropped from 7.04 to 3.56 between 1800 and 1900;[44] by 2016 the number fell further to approximately 1.8.[45]

A decrease in average family size has not, however, corresponded to a de-emphasis of the biological family model. Legally, biology continues to play a significant role in how the United States constructs what is or is not a family. Child Protective Services, for instance, currently—if not historically—makes it a priority to reunify biological families as opposed to advocating first for adoption or permanent foster care placement, working from the assumption that children are best off with their blood relatives—provided that they can offer basic safety and developmental needs.[46] State governments provide services to biologically based parents to help strengthen their ability to care for their children instead of immediately advocating for permanent resettlement of offspring. Such a strategy suggests a hierarchy that ranks biological families above other forms, and it implies an essential basis to the concept of family that is rooted not in relationships between parent and child but in the genetic link established at conception. Legal opposition to same-sex unions also used an argument that privileged the biological family, proposing that gay or lesbian couples should not be allowed to marry precisely because they could not reproduce. This logic presupposes that biological connections determined who was part of a family; otherwise the argument could be nullified with the objection that a same-sex couple could establish a family through adoption. It also assumed that the concept of family must include children in the first place.[47]

These examples are indicative of an overarching American assumption that a couple must have biological children to become a "family." A casual observation of other areas of American life reinforce this assumption: couples without children talk about how they plan to "start a family," as if their own relationship is somehow insufficient to be termed familial and requires the presence of biological children to fulfill it. Holidays, arguably the most collectively esteemed of vacation days, are often spent with biological family members, even though one might vastly prefer to spend the day with friends. End-of-life practices in American culture also indicate privileges given to biological family members, as Americans tend to purchase mausoleums or grave plots for the purpose of being laid to rest beside blood relatives. Likewise, it is blood relatives who occupy the first row at the funeral, and blood relatives who typically receive the deceased's inheritance. These examples reinforce that the word "family" means shared blood, a finding that sociological research supports. Research found that 45.3 percent of Americans define the term *family* as a heterosexual couple with children, with approximately 33 percent of this group explicitly mentioning the presence of biological children as the factor that determines whether a configuration of individuals constitutes a family.[48] For these individuals, children's genes matter. They concretize the union between spouses and create an inseparable bond between adults and children alike.[49] There is, from this point of view, something superior about the relationship between biological children and their parents that cannot be replicated without the genetic link, and consequentially, this produces a hierarchy of nurturing relationships that ranks biological families above other relational configurations. Same-sex couples, single individuals, or heterosexual couples who adopt or use reproductive technology in which one participant is not genetically related to the child may all in the end function as nuclear units in which adults raise children; these units do not, however, qualify as families according to this 33 percent of participants.[50]

To define family in such a way implies a commitment to certain essentialist arguments about identity: men and women may be said to have specific roles in reproduction determined by biology that are expected to be used in the way that God or nature intended them to be used. The man provides sperm, and the woman provides the egg and a womb. Sexual intercourse allows for the joining of sperm and egg into a zygote that eventually forms into an infant who is subsequently born from the mother's womb, thereby allowing both her and the male involved to announce that yes, they *have* started their family and by so doing have attained the titles of mother and father that put them at the pinnacle of the relational pyramid.[51] Under this construction, then, the inability to reproduce signals a fault in the natural order—a woman's body is supposed to be able to carry a child, just as a man's should be able to offer sperm to the cause—and while it may be pushing too far to say that the grief that derives from infertility or reproductive loss emerges from a construction such as this, such assumptions about what it means to have a properly functioning body could certainly make the processing of such events more difficult.

In contrast to the 45 percent of Americans who espouse something of an essentialist view of the biological group, 29 percent of Americans acknowledge that adoptive children might be part of the biological family, though they do so reluctantly. As one participant in a sociological study explained, "There have to be children involved or marriage [for it to be a family]. . . . If there's no kids and they're not married, that doesn't, to me—there needs to be either marriage or some kind of blood relation for that to be a family."[52] However, later in that same interview, the participant began to shift her position to include adoptive children into the family structure when she said, "Not that there couldn't be a wonderful family adoption thing going on. . . . I guess I consider [adoptive children and parents] a family, even though that's not a blood relative."[53] It is worth noting here that the participant included adopted children with hesitancy—as indicated by the phrase "I guess"—and that this inclusion seemed to be the exception to the norm—as indicated by the phrase "even though." In sum, of this group it might be said that yes, alternatives to biology count as real family units; that they are included, however, is not the same as saying they are ideal.

What the first two groups in this study—which total 74.6 percent of the participants—reveal is at least a degree of commitment to the primacy of the biological family, to blood relations, and perhaps to essentialist commitments to gendered identity. This image of the family contrasts with that of the remaining 25.4 percent of Americans whom researchers term "inclusionists." Of this group, only 1 percent mentioned children at all as a factor defining families. Relationships between partners transcended all other factors in this cohort, including blood relations, and nontraditional structures including same-sex unions and platonic friendships counted as families. The relational connection between individuals therefore became the root of what a family was.[54]

Collective evidence from across the social sciences indicates that approximately 75 percent of Americans tend to prize the biological family model over others, causing individuals to operate within a cultural script that generates a certain set of expectations that may affect their outlook as they begin to contemplate starting families of their own. However, it may also be that the primacy afforded to blood relationships is beginning to shift: the changing contours of marriage, the role of women outside the home, and increased life expectancy are all factors that contribute to an evolving cultural mindset of what a family is and what it looks like. Likewise, the Supreme Court's decision to overturn the Defense of Marriage Act and the increasing number of corporations offering benefits to unmarried domestic partners are just two examples of an evolution in the American definition of family. Indeed, it may well be that further transformations in American society will press up against assumptions about the word in years to come.[55]

However, while the aforementioned factors in the United States may indeed be gradually shifting the supremacy of the biological family model, it is still an assumed model for many. Cultural assumptions about what a family is, therefore, can clash against the biological realities of those whose bodies cannot reproduce.[56] This may be, somewhat ironically, more surprising for heterosexual couples—who tend to be perceived as the bedrock of "family" in the United States—than it is for others. In cases where individuals are either single or have partners of the same sex, they may know earlier—before experiences of infertility or reproductive loss—that an additional party such as a surrogate, a mother placing her child for adoption, or a gamete donor is needed in order for them to undertake a parental role. A single man, for instance, or a gay couple simply does not have a uterus in which to grow a baby. Likewise, a single woman or lesbian couple lacks sperm. However, heterosexual couples may enter into the procreative process assuming that they can carry their own children, that conception is easy, and that reproduction is a private matter to be undertaken beneath the sheets of one's bed. In this way, heterosexual couples emblematize the self-sufficiency that Americans tend to pride themselves on: only heterosexual couples have the luxury of believing that they can make a baby all by themselves and, because all others are excluded from the process of procreation, that this baby is theirs alone. Through a diagnosis of infertility or the experience of reproductive loss, however, they may discover that this belief in reproductive autonomy is but an illusion.

The Primacy of the Biological Family and Its Significance for Infertility and Reproductive Loss

The reproductive technology industry flourishes in the United States, indicating a societal craving for biological children that perpetuates the biological as the privileged family model. Rhetoric of "family values" furthers this craving, connoting that biological families structured in a certain way are not only desirable but also ground the basic health and well-being of American society. The proper adult life, therefore, becomes one in which marriage and parenthood—preferably biological parenthood—materialize: one might even go so far as to say biological family functions as an idol in the United States.[57]

Yet other forms of family exist—including foster parenting, adoption, and childless living—so it becomes possible to question whether the biological family is indeed a superior form of family, even the essence of family, or whether it is merely constructed as such. To query whether the biological family is a construct of family instead of its essence, however, may be to question the very definition of family itself. If the word *family* means anything, it would seem at first to signify those relationships marked by a genetic link. After the fall, for instance, Adam and Eve did not adopt children; they birthed them. Indeed, the perpetuation of the human race depends on biological reproduction, to such an extent that to question the biological family seems to question the very existence of humanity.

And yet linking genes from a man and woman together is not the only prerequisite for the development of human life, for while an ovum and sperm are both necessary for the creation of a baby, so is a uterus. That uterus houses the product of conception from its earliest stages through birth; it becomes the flexible space that allows the zygote an opportunity to develop a spinal cord, brain, arms, legs, eyes, and all its other parts. It nurtures the developing fetus by delivering food and providing a place to rest. The woman who achieves a wanted pregnancy, therefore, embarks upon a relational contract with the developing infant to keep it safe, fed, and flourishing. While the joining of sperm and egg creates a ball of cells, that ball of cells alone is not enough for the creation of human life—the gestational space is also a requirement.[58]

If the defining factor of *family* were the relationship developed during gestation—or even after—then the genetic connection with one's child would be of less consequence, and thus both adoption and traditional surrogacy arrangements might be more desirable forms of reproduction. In the United States, however, traditional surrogacy is almost nonexistent, and when individuals adopt, the question of who the "real parents" are may linger because of the assumption that parenthood is defined by genetics.[59] The existence of birth parents may therefore be a cause of stress or confusion for adoptive parents or even a perceived threat to the adoptive parents' integrity; such reactions are another indicator of the role genes play in understanding what a "real family" is in the United States.[60]

The value of genetics in the construction of the American family therefore suggests a privileging of DNA over relationship, which might also be said to signal a devaluing of the unique contribution women can offer to reproduction—namely, a relationship with the developing infant. One might counter that women also contribute genetic material; however, this line of reasoning compounds rather than alleviates the inequality when one considers the history and significance of knowledge of "the seed." For hundreds of years, Western societies assumed only male sperm contributed to genetic reproduction, with the existence of the human female ovum remaining undiscovered until the late 1920s. As a result, men sought to control women's bodies in order to control the seed: practices such as supervised courting, the assurance of virginity at marriage, and the prohibition against extramarital affairs all benefited men, ensuring that they could claim offspring as theirs.

The discovery of the ovum transformed the significance of women's role in reproduction. The historical belief was that that men contributed the "seed" while women contributed the womb or relationship with the developing infant to the reproductive process. But when scientists discovered the role of the ovum in reproduction, what emerged was not only the elevation of a woman's genetic contribution but also a devaluation of pregnancy and the embodied relationship that a woman—by nature of carrying the pregnancy—can develop with the fetus over the course of nine months. In other words, women lost the opportunity to champion their own reproductive contributions by claiming the privileges given to men's form of involvement in the process. The increased awareness of women's biological contributions to reproduction and its subsequent validation of the privilege afforded the biological family thus did little to respond to the degradation of the relationships that form the foundation of pregnancy, which in turn meant that it did little to uphold women's unique contribution to family creation. As a result, when women became able to define parenthood through genetics alone, they did not achieve liberation from a patriarchal view of reproduction but rather came to abide within it.[61]

A related objection would be this: the discovery that women contributed the ovum led to an awareness of the genetic role that women play in reproduction, but this awareness validated women through a source of their own oppression. To equate a woman's role in reproduction with a source of her own oppression might be seen as a far less dramatic example of freeing slaves and then allowing them to become slaveholders. In both scenarios, the overarching worldview remains, even if members of the formerly oppressed class can now claim to benefit from it. Justifying the genetic primacy of families through the logic of "women can do it too" therefore justifies a woman's role in reproduction by fashioning her into the image of a man. It does not, however, justify her role by validating the contribution historically believed to be hers alone.

Consequences of Biological Family Primacy for Surrogacy

The desire for a genetic connection to one's children almost inevitably factors into the decision to choose reproductive technology over adoption. Indeed, perhaps the most compelling data to reinforce that assertion is this: demand for surrogates in the United States far outpaces availability while the number of children seeking families—especially in the foster care system—outpaces the desire of potential parents to adopt them. Particularly in relation to the foster care system, this may be because children are older, have developmental needs that parents are uncertain they have the resources to handle, or have concerns the birth parents will be able to reclaim guardianship. However, intended parents may well feel hesitant to adopt out of the foster system precisely because there is not enough societal support for them to do so: stigmas against children with special needs, a sense that older kids are already too "damaged" by the system for parents to make a positive impact, and general confusion about the role of birth parents all act as deterrents. Such factors may lead intended parents to desire the imaginary child who does not yet exist but who hypothetically shares their eye color, their hair texture, their intelligence quota, their love of football, or their peanut allergy more than they desire the living, breathing child whose body, whose smile, and whose personality currently exists, only it does not resemble theirs. The former child, after all, offers reliability through the presence of shared genes, giving parents a concrete, though possibly illusory, sense of what to expect for their future—whereas the non-genetically related child is unknown in all regards. An adult considering adopting out of the foster system may worry that a given child could be genetically predisposed to substance abuse, psychological instability, or other factors that might have been passed on by their genetic parents, who presumably had something wrong with them or the child would not have been in the foster system in the first place. Such a child, under this belief system, is damaged by their genetic heritage, and as a result, the infertile parents may reason, the child who could be fashioned in their genetic image is the safer bet because it is the one over which they theoretically have a greater degree of control.[62] The genetic tie, therefore, becomes a desirable prerequisite for perceived reproductive success in the United States in a way that relationship does not.

Indeed, it is possible to quantify the value placed on genes over the value placed on relationship in the United States by considering the compensation offered to egg donors and surrogates. Egg donors make, on average, about $8,000 per donation, which is roughly the equivalent of $23.81 per hour for an approximately two-week cycle.[63] In contrast, surrogates in the United States are paid on average $45,000 over a forty-week period, averaging $6.53 per hour.[64] This data indicates that surrogates receive three and a half times less per hour than donors do, presumably because the value of carrying a child is less than the value of providing genes for one. Equally striking when considering this data are the criteria used to choose a donor versus a surrogate. Those with the means to use assisted reproduction pick egg donors primarily for characteristics linked to genes, including skin, hair, and eye color. They desire donors who resemble them in some way, which means that more often than not, donors are high achievers, are white, and perhaps share a love of music or sports. In short, intended parents tend to choose donors who are like themselves to some degree so that donors' instrumental value corresponds to intended parents'. That is part of the point, after all, to find the genes that most mimic one's own; otherwise adoption might be more of a consideration. In contrast, intended parents choose a surrogate primarily by her track record of how successfully her body executed pregnancies in the past (and most clinics prohibit women who have not given birth from being surrogates). Where SAT scores matter for egg donors, the number of babies birthed matters for surrogates, and as a result, surrogates tend to be poorer and less educated than donors and are also more likely to be minorities.[65] Phrased more concretely, it is more acceptable for a poor woman to carry a rich woman's baby than it is for a poor woman to provide a rich woman with ova. Likewise, it is more acceptable for a black woman to carry a white woman's baby than it is for a white woman to choose a black egg donor. Surrogacy practices therefore symbolize that there are insiders and outsiders in reproduction, individuals with reproductive power and individuals without, individuals who belong, even tangentially, in the family and individuals who, by virtue of their genetics, do not.

Conclusion

Those who have the resources to hire surrogates in the United States tend to be upper class and white, which means that it is those views of family that affect the choices intended parents make. Within other segments of American society, it may be that the biological family bears less primacy than it does among those who have the power to orchestrate reproduction through the use of technology. However, nonwhite Americans are also more likely to lack access to reproductive technology and therefore have less influence on how it operates. Surrogacy in the United States, therefore, is not only an industry but a politics that may be said to operate in the service of orchestrating white, upper-class reproduction, of allowing privilege to reproduce privilege. The tragedy, however, is that this is not what surrogacy necessarily seeks to do: virtually any surrogate arrangement emerges from loss, so the possibility of reproduction via the surrogate becomes an opportunity for theodicy to conclude, for an evil to find redemption, for a surd to obtain meaning. This is what intended parents ultimately seek—a child who will provide the conclusion to their reproductive narrative and who will write an ending to their own suffering. If they privilege a child who looks like them and bears their genes in the process, if they perceive the surrogate as someone with whom they have a business arrangement rather than as a friend or family member, then this may say more about the power of privileged societal values than about the parents themselves—indeed, parents might well make different reproductive choices if different factors shaped their beliefs. Surrogacy in the United States consequently has the possibility to exploit the loss of intended parents in ways that perpetuate the primacy given to the biological family, ensuring that society's most privileged have the opportunity to reproduce and that patriarchal, genetically based views of family persist, all the while affecting the politics of reproduction in ways that extend beyond the individual's actual desires and into society at large.

The traumas of reproductive loss and infertility instantiate physical and existential crises within the human psyche, and if one assumes that humans have the capacity to exercise free will, then it follows that those who experience reproductive loss—regardless of race, economics, or other factors—may find meaning in and move forward from the aftermath of these events via a path of their own choosing. However, unspoken assumptions about what it means to inhabit the sphere of family within the cultural construct that exists in the United States hold power over what appears to be freely chosen. This embedded construct affects not only the choice to use a surrogate but also the exercise of the surrogacy experience itself, creating a vicious cycle, with family practices affecting societal norms and societal norms, in turn, perpetuating family practices. American surrogacy practices, therefore, may say more about the overarching values of those with power in the United States than they say about the essence of surrogacy itself.

2

Surrogacy as Culturally Constructed

Surrogates are elusive; they are category evaders. They are not supposed to be mothers, yet they bear children. They are workers, yet the product emerges from their own bodies instead of sliding off a conveyer belt.[1] They could be likened to singers and actors, both of whom use their bodies to create something exterior to themselves—a song, a character. Yet these latter professions exist in the realm of the enviable. Tabloids and television shows dedicate themselves to dissecting the glamour of the pop star and the makeup of the celebrity so that those who do not dwell in their world can participate in it from afar. They are the stuff of childhood fantasies, of toddlers in oversized boas and high heels, parading across a worn scarlet towel that stands in for a red carpet. That same toddler would probably not imagine herself a surrogate. It lacks the glamour.

Ironically, while the allure of the celebrity singer or actor is partially the sexiness of their bodies, it is the sexed nature of surrogacy that renders it taboo. A woman carrying the baby of a man who is not her husband seems dangerously close to adultery. A woman paid to carry that baby seems ill bred because babies should be born of love, not birthed for money, and a woman willing to give up a baby appears to lack the capacity to bond with the fetus that every woman is supposed to possess.[2] The surrogate is therefore an antithesis of culturally normative views of womanhood, her actions pressing against accepted expectations about women's identity and the kind of relationships presumed to exist between them, the men who marry them, and the children who emerge from their bodies. Like prostitutes, they use their bodies to meet primal needs—the need for sex, the need for children—and in so doing, they become sites of a culturally taboo, and therefore distasteful, economy in which those who have the means may pay to achieve their own gratification, be it the gratification of experiencing an orgasm or the gratification of holding an infant in one's arms.

And yet, even as the surrogate contrasts with stereotyped womanhood, she is also the embodiment of a successful theodicy, for what her body holds within it is the curative to the reproductive trauma experienced by the intended parents. She can make good on their losses. She can manifest their dreams, and when she is successful in her charge, their reproductive story receives its ending, and their suffering receives its meaning.

When casually considered, however, the most prominent surrogates tend to be more tendentious than superheroic. Hagar from Genesis or Offred from *The Handmaid's Tale* each present troubled views of surrogates as women who struggle to integrate in their relationships with the intended parents and who are seen as slaves, second-class citizens, or objects. How much stories such as these reflect the current realities of surrogacy is hard to say without an examination of modern practices. Such an examination reveals variety at both individual and cross-cultural levels. To illustrate the commonalities and distinctions, then, what follows is an overview of surrogacy in the contexts of the United States, India, and Israel.

Who Is the American Surrogate?

The average surrogate in the United States is a working class, white, Christian, twenty-seven-year-old high school graduate, married with three children.[3] Ninety-eight percent of surrogates state that they are not planning to have any more children of their own, and approximately 30 percent are homemakers. Those who work outside the home tend to hold jobs in the service industry.[4] Some state they are motivated by empathy for infertile couples, that they enjoy pregnancy itself, or that they hope their participation in the creation of new life will assuage their guilt from a prior abortion or from putting up one of their own children for adoption.[5] Most view surrogacy as a calling or vocation regardless of their motivations, and they report that they had an interest in helping infertile couples procreate long before they knew surrogacy existed.

Anthropological studies of surrogates in the United States reveal that they often state altruistic motives and discredit the role that payment might play in their decision. Helena Ragoné postulates that the negative cognitions surrounding compensation serve dual functions: First, they allow the surrogate to show that she agrees with the cultural assumption that children are priceless. To be able to provide a child to a couple is immeasurable, unquantifiable in terms of its value, such that there is no dollar amount that could equate.[6] Second, it reinforces the surrogate's tendency to perceive her participation in terms of gift giving rather than product production, which in turn translates into a specific way of viewing her relationship with the intended parents.[7] The surrogate would be an employee of the couple were she producing a product for them, thereby relegating her to a subservient position; however, as a gift giver, she assumes a locus of power, for it is she who possesses what is desirable—a functioning womb.

The surrogate also often perceives herself as participating in a relational contract—an agreement rooted in the cultivation of relationships—as opposed to a business contract predicated on the exchange of services or goods. Her commitment to relationship allows her to hold the belief that her relationship with the parents will last indefinitely, perhaps functioning as a form of resistance against clinics and intended parents, who may impress that the relationship is intended to last only for the duration of the pregnancy. The surrogate, however, maintains that the child that she births creates a link between herself and the parents that endures precisely because of the existence of the child. The child, after all, could not exist without her body to gestate it, and therefore to erase her from the narrative of the child's life would be to erase the child itself. Even if intended parents keep the surrogate's existence a secret, they know, and the surrogate knows, the child's origins. The child therefore functions as a permanent link between the intended parents and the surrogate, and that link, that relationship, far exceeds in value whatever payment the surrogate receives. Indeed, the exchange of money may arguably function as an attempt to reduce surrogacy to a business contract and to invalidate the grounding role of relationships.[8] This is not to say that surrogates should not be paid, but it is to say that money's role holds power in the interpretation of the surrogate's role.

Class and Power Divides in Third-Party Relationships

In a chart describing twenty-eight American heterosexual intended-parent couples provided by Helena Ragoné, all the fathers and all but two of the wives had higher education degrees, and the average family salary for these couples exceeded $100,000.[9] In contrast, in a similar chart of twenty-eight surrogates, the average income of married surrogates was $38,700 and the average income of unmarried surrogates ranged from $16,000 to $24,000.[10] Of these women, five had a college degree, one had an associate's degree, and the remainder had a high school education or less. Ragoné's data illustrates that surrogates usually lack their intended parents' financial privilege, an almost universal trend in surrogacy arrangements.[11] Intended parents have money to pay for surrogacy; surrogates are usually not affluent enough to hire a surrogate themselves.

Some programs allow surrogates and intended parents to remain anonymous from one another in order to mitigate relational difficulties most efficiently; in these closed programs, intended parents and surrogates avoid contact in order to negate the possibility that one or the other might misuse their own relational power—in other words, to avoid another Baby M. case. The creation of life here might be said to be reduced to a purely business transaction instead of any kind of relational contract in these scenarios because these programs effectively terminate social engagement by preventing embodied knowledge of the other. The surrogate may be whomever the parents imagine her to be, and likewise the reverse. Neither need speak with the other, which also means that neither need engage in confrontation with the other. Indeed, at the conclusion of anonymous surrogacy, the only evidence of the connection between all parties is the child itself.[12]

Not all surrogate arrangements are anonymous in the United States, however. Some agencies encourage the surrogate and intended parents to meet, write letters, and jointly attend the birth. They may also employ scripting techniques to help participants create boundaries around their relationships during this process, with Ragoné observing that programs frame the surrogate's work in ways that mitigate the most preponderant fear among both intended parents and professionals: that surrogates will try to keep the baby. Surrogacy agencies therefore provide tools to structure the surrogate's experience so that she feels prepared to part with the infant at its birth. Foremost, they encourage surrogates to believe that they are women with great responsibility, the responsibility to carry and birth a child for individuals who cannot do so themselves. Programs also impress empathy for intended parents on the surrogate to combat any temptation the surrogate may have to keep the child. Intended parents yearn for children, they say. They yearn for biological children, and because of that, their own experiences of infertility or reproductive loss before deciding on surrogacy caused untold suffering. Agencies accordingly make sure the surrogate understands that she provides the last hope for the dream that intended parents have yet to realize, and they remind her that her body is able to achieve what the intended parents' cannot: the birth of a soft-skinned, cooing infant.[13] Hers is the body they need to write the happy ending to their reproductive story, and if she tries to keep the child her body cultivates, then she will inflict a final, devastating emotional wound.

Agencies also rely on the assumption that biological children are desirable in order to convince the surrogate that it is appropriate to part with the infant—because she is not genetically related to the baby, it is not her own. Likewise, parents will be hurt by her decision to keep the baby precisely because they are—in cases where their egg and sperm were utilized—the genetic parents and therefore the rightful parents. This assumption that genetics determines parenthood tends to be shared by intended parents and surrogates alike. Reproductive loss or infertility previously instantiated suffering for intended parents because the good that was desired—the biological child—could not be manifested. Likewise, most surrogates believe that biological children are a good worth having, in part because they are a good they already achieved and in which they found value. Parenthood has been a meaningful experience for the surrogate, an experience she wants others to share, and as a result, agencies can draw on the surrogate's assumption about the value of biological children and use it to achieve their desired end: the successful transfer of the baby. For if the surrogate realizes just how valuable a biological child is to its genetic parents, then she will be willing to part with this gestational offspring—to which she has no biological connection—so that intended parents can have the experience of raising it. To that end, the surrogate herself may subscribe to the belief that genetics and not gestation define parenthood and may believe that the business contract she signed should be privileged above the relationship with the fetus she developed during the pregnancy.

Along with responsibility, programs also impress that surrogates have great power because intended parents could not achieve their dream of parenthood without them. The surrogate therefore functions as a woman with a mission or a calling to create biologically based parents and is nothing short of a hero. Agencies reinforce this narrative by impressing upon surrogates that they are unique and special and that they can achieve the impossible. They encourage surrogates to construct their experience in a way that negates economic power, for although intended parents may have the funds to pay for surrogacy, only the body of the surrogate can do this particular work. Only her body can create life; only her volition can give that baby over to the intended parents; only her desire has the potential to devastate them one last time if she tries to keep the infant. The ultimate power, therefore, lies with the surrogate herself to create not just a life but a lifetime of happiness or a lifetime of loss.[14]

In structuring the narrative that the surrogate uses to define her experience, programs claim that she has both great responsibility and great power. Yet what goes unstated is the program's power; it is the program that structures how the surrogate understands her own experience and the program that claims to give authority to surrogates while simultaneously being directive. Even a well-intentioned attempt to script the surrogate's experience robs her of a degree of interpretive agency by encouraging her to see the experience from a singular perspective, the perspective of the agency, which in turn mirrors the priorities of the intended parents who pay the fees. Hence, the surrogate is to privilege the suffering of intended parents over any desire she might have because a contract is a contract, a deal is a deal. If a surrogate said she would give the baby up, then that is what she must do, regardless of what feels right to her, because the suffering of the parents is simply too great to contemplate the alternative.

At best, surrogacy programs use adaptive strategies that will make the imminent separation of surrogate and infant easier for all involved parties. At worst, however, the narrative they encourage surrogates to construct might be considered a form of social coercion, wherein they write her reproductive narrative for her, reducing the creation of life to a business contract for the purpose of ensuring that the product—here, the baby—efficiently and successfully reaches the hands of those with economic power—in this case, the intended parents. The relational dimension among parents, surrogates, and third parties thereby becomes subservient.

The Surrogate as Power Holder

Policies such as these raise the question of whether the mechanisms used by programs to develop healthy relationships between third parties and intended parents actually impinge on the surrogate's agency and interpretation of the experience. Yet surrogates are far from powerless. Even as the surrogate finds herself in a subservient position, she simultaneously holds power because of her body's fertility and also because so few women desire the job. The demand for a surrogate outweighs the supply in both the United States and abroad, with demand increasing, especially as a surrogate can now be employed by not only infertile heterosexual couples but also same-sex couples, transgender couples, and single intended parents who may require their assistance in order to become biologically based parents. The sheer need for the surrogate's existence, therefore, gives her a substantial degree of influence, so that from the vantage of the agency and intended parents, the surrogate is a valuable commodity, and her fertility bears a power that trumps whatever wealth the parents may have. This is a belief acknowledged both by intended parents and by the surrogate, who is often aware that her ultimate strength lies in her ability to provide what those who contract with her lack and desperately desire—children.[15] Babies, therefore, become her leverage, functioning in parallel to intended parents' financial resources so that just as intended parents may withhold payment if the surrogate does not meet the agreed-upon contractual demands, so the surrogate can withhold the use of her womb or the resulting infant. The surrogate's fertility can thus function both benevolently and as a source of exploitation, just as money can for the intended parents. This means that the greatest resource of the surrogate—her womb and the baby she can create in it—is also her greatest weapon, such that the surrogate may perceive herself as having just as much power as intended parents do, instead of seeing herself as an object of exploitation.

Communication Trends in American Surrogacy

The surrogate's power is also facilitated by agencies that structure the perceptions of intended parents: they may encourage intended parents to write letters to the surrogate, call her, go with her to doctor's visits, and in cases where surrogates are local, attend a Lamaze class or the delivery itself. The intended father may cut the umbilical cord as a sign of the severing connection between the surrogate and baby, and after the birth, programs may instruct intended parents to offer a gift to the surrogate in thanks for her efforts.[16] In addition, they may tell intended parents to avoid arguing in front of the surrogate, encouraging them instead to present an image of a healthy marriage and an ideal home in which to welcome an infant. They may also tell intended parents to avoid discussing topics where their beliefs may differ from a surrogate's on tendentious issues that tangentially relate to surrogacy—such as abortion and whether a mother should work outside the home—so that intended parents can prevent conflict.[17]

Programs' scripting of the relationship between intended parents and surrogates continues after the birth of the infant. Programs may strongly suggest that surrogates and intended parents terminate their relationship after the birth occurs, or keep their communication to a minimum. This process is often easier for intended parents than it is for surrogates: while some surrogates are happy to reduce contact to a yearly holiday card or to cease contact entirely, others come to view the couple as friends, so that the contact elimination that the agency suggests comes across to the surrogate as contrary to her expectations of the relationship. In contrast, intended parents often have an easier time terminating the relationship because they no longer need the surrogate's assistance.[18] The contract is complete; she has handed over the child to its rightful owners.[19]

The connection between intended parents and surrogate may also diminish after the infant's birth in other ways if parents choose to keep the use of third-party reproduction a secret from their family, friends, and the resulting child, with the goal of maintaining the illusion that the procedures were not used. While it is difficult to quantify how often surrogate children are not told of their origins, Ragoné cites examples of parents who do just that—an adoptive mother who fakes nine months of pregnancy and childbirth; a father who appears unannounced at a program director's home, demanding his file and stating that he had not made an appointment because he wanted to ensure the program did not have time to make copies; a mother who, while still waiting for the surrogate to deliver, tells Ragoné she may not tell the child about its origins so as to avoid admitting that she is infertile.[20]

Parents who do not disclose the use of a surrogate reflect the more documented tendency of those in the United States to refrain from telling children about their origins when their conception arises from egg, sperm, or embryo donation. It also reflects the historical trend of not telling adopted children of their origins. Privacy concerns, fears that the lack of a genetic relationship or knowledge about one's genetic makeup would upset the child, that it would threaten the identity of the parents, that the knowledge would disrupt relationships between the parents and the child, or that the information is irrelevant because parenthood is a relational contract and not a biological one all determine parents' decision not to disclose.[21] Parents' own cognitions about the egg or sperm donor—when one is used—may also contribute, as may the general power of the biological family as the preferred family form.[22]

While parents may already be inclined not to disclose this information to their children for a number of reasons, nondisclosure may be further reinforced by ingrained American medical practices. Individual doctors may not necessarily enforce the American Society for Reproductive Medicine's guideline to encourage disclosure or keep records of which donor, if one is used, contributed genetic material to specific parents, thereby implying that such knowledge is not a priority or a good worth preserving.[23] As a result, such practices of omission reinforce the desire of intended parents to privilege the biological family or, in this case, the illusion of the biological family. If donors cannot be traced, if it is possible to erase their involvement from the reproductive narrative, then perhaps intended parents can construct a story of parenthood that removes the third party entirely so that they can effectually validate themselves within the boundaries of the biological family model. To that end, studies find that children conceived via these procedures are less likely to be told of their origins than children brought into a family via adoption; however, like the trajectory of adoption—where disclosure rates were historically low but have been recently on the rise—it is becoming more common for American parents to disclose third-party use.[24]

Pragmatically, it is more difficult to attempt to erase a surrogate's involvement in reproduction than it is to erase a gamete donor's, yet the underlying justification for so doing may be said to be the same in each circumstance: it privileges the intended parents' goals for fitting into the societal norm of biological parenthood. It solidifies their parental power by eradicating any potential competition for the title of "parent." Yet what benefits the parent does not necessarily benefit the surrogate or the child. Practices that acknowledge the surrogate—like gift giving or thank-you notes—are often crucial to the surrogate's own quest to find meaning and satisfaction from the process.[25] Moreover, psychological research demonstrates that children who are not told of their origins through third-party reproduction at an early age subsequently experience themselves as different from the family who raised them, while teenagers and adults who discover that they were conceived with donated genetic material can experience a number of detrimental cognitions and feelings, including mistrust, abandonment by medical professionals who advocated nondisclosure, and a sense of frustration or loss when they cannot obtain donor information.[26] These studies mirror the findings of individuals who were not told of their origins through adoption.[27] In both cases, finding out that one's origins were not as they seemed reveals itself as a form of identity betrayal. The assumptions that such individuals developed about their familial history, their genetic propensity for certain illnesses, those qualities they assumed were "inherited" from the people who raised them—a passion for music, perhaps, or a dislike of green squash—turn out to be falsehoods. What remains is the knowledge that one was lied to, that relationships had false foundations, and that those same relationships, which appeared to root aspects of identity, never existed in the way that had been constructed.[28]

While data about disclosure rates remains difficult to come by for surrogacy, the cases that document it reveal that some couples feel they need surrogates in order to establish their identity as biologically based parents, yet in order to maintain their status or identity as such, they must hide the existence of the surrogate. Such parents thus appear to undermine their own argument, for the practice of secrecy belies their belief that they are not in fact real parents because the use of the surrogate precludes that. By keeping a child's origins secret, it would seem as if parents are trying to present a fertile self to the world at the expense of both the child, to whom they lie either actively or through omission, and the surrogate, whose crucial role in creating life they no longer acknowledge.[29]

Such scenarios—however common or rare—also reveal the irony that the traumas of reproductive loss or infertility that inaugurate crises of identity in intended parents can in turn lead to identity crises and trauma in the next generation. Procedures designed to allow parents to adhere to the biological family model—when used without openness—may indeed allow parents to hold to the illusion that authentic family is the biological family, but they also necessitate that children navigate the fallout of that assumption for their own identity, a journey made increasingly problematic when one is raised without with an honest understanding of one's origins. The trauma of one generation thereby conveys to the next.

These secretive practices may occur, in part, because of the societal stigma that intended parents feel accompanies their inability to carry life to term.[30] The primacy of the biological family model, in other words, pressures parents to find a way to identify themselves within it. It may also arise because of the very real pain that accompanies their experience of not being able to easily create a family, as the previous chapter described. Even so, attempts to protect the parents may in turn have negative consequences for those who participate in surrogacy.

An analysis of domestic surrogacy practices such as this one inevitably raises the question of the degree to which they are culturally constructed or essentially delineated. Tangentially, it queries whether agencies promote best practices among participants, circumscribing relationships to make the process as fulfilling as possible, or whether they promote practices that benefit the power players. It therefore becomes essential to consider surrogacy in cultures outside the United States to understand what happens domestically. In other words, considering the beliefs and practices in other contexts may illuminate the assumptions that drive domestic ones.

The Cost of Assisted Reproduction and Why Americans Use Indian Surrogates

Surrogacy in the United States is not inexpensive, nor is it a simple process to undertake. Legal restrictions vary by state, creating confusion as to who allows what. Arizona, for instance, bans all surrogacy; Louisiana bans traditional surrogacy; and in the state of Washington, surrogacy is legal, but a surrogate cannot receive compensation. As a result, intended parents who investigate surrogacy in the United States face a complicated array of laws and regulations, sometimes in addition to paying for either themselves or the surrogate to travel to a state where the procedures are legal.[31]

Surrogacy expenses add to the logistical burdens. The cost for one cycle hovers between $50,000 and $100,000 (including payment to the surrogate as well as medical procedure fees), exorbitant for the average American. Although some rely on insurance to help, many insurers do not cover all treatment options.[32] However, even if the intended parents are working with an insurer that covers treatments, some fertility clinics do not take insurance. Some intended parents are able to apply to their insurance company for reimbursement or use the flexible-spending programs their insurance companies provide, but others finance the procedures by depleting their savings accounts, borrowing money from relatives, dipping into their 401(k) or other retirement savings, taking out a home equity loan or second mortgage, or taking on credit card debt. Additionally, some clinics provide financing programs to help intended parents pay for their procedures.

The cost of surrogacy remains prohibitive for many in the United States even with financing options, rendering it a technology that primarily exists for the wealthy and causing surrogacy to function as a luxury item in the United States. However, the desire for surrogate reproduction is not limited to the wealthy, so the financial and legal inaccessibility creates a void between what Americans desire and what they can obtain. Americans have turned to medical tourism to find alternatives, primarily but not exclusively in India, which until 2017 met the needs of these Americans in several regards. First, the full cost of surrogacy hovers around $15,000 in India, a fraction of the cost in the United States, even with airfare to and from the country. In addition, the Indian government did not intervene in the burgeoning surrogate industry until after 2015. The absence of laws determining what could or could not happen in surrogacy arrangements meant that surrogates lacked any legal precedent to keep the infant they carried, unlike in the United States, where many states have laws granting surrogates varying degrees of parental rights. This appealed to intended parents who worried their surrogate might lay claim to the child, as Mary Beth Whitehead did.[33] The lack of governmental oversight also led parents to believe that they could maintain greater control of the pregnancy than they might have if the surrogate lived in the United States.[34] Intended parents could pay for surrogates to live in supervised housing, regulate women's diets by paying a supplement for healthy meals, and pay workers to monitor surrogates to ensure they were not smoking during the pregnancy. The ability of intended parents to regulate the surrogate's body—and to do so at a lower price point—made surrogacy in India an attractive option to those in the United States, especially those who could not afford domestic surrogacy.[35]

Characteristics of Indian Surrogacy

While surrogates across cultures tend to be poorer and less educated than the intended parents for whom they carry children, the disparity in India is particularly marked. Amrita Pande found that the education of an Indian surrogate ranges from illiterate to a high school diploma, with the mean somewhere in the middle school years. Surrogates are almost always financially destitute—with an average income of $50 per month—and married, and it is not atypical for their husbands to be unemployed or underemployed. Surrogacy therefore offers a substantial cash influx that is the equivalent of roughly five years of income from other jobs they might have attained.[36] Many possess lofty dreams of how the approximately $5,000 payment will transform their lives, and they imagine the possibility of a home, better schools for their children, or a new business for their husband. However, Pande notes that most mothers do not achieve long-term economic betterment because they were surrogates.[37] Pande also reports that many surrogates dream of long-term relationships with the intended parents and believe that they will shower them with gifts for their own children or help them immigrate to the intended parents' countries; these dreams rarely materialize.

Pande's ethnography emphasizes that intended parents and doctors seek control over surrogates even as surrogates practice forms of resistance. All surrogates live either within the clinic itself or in a nearby hostel, both of which are monitored twenty-four hours a day. Within the clinic—which houses the women perceived to be more difficult to manage—women sleep eight to a room in single iron beds decorated with photographs of Lord Krishna and healthy babies. They are not permitted to use the stairs and cannot operate the elevator without assistance from the clinic staff; most spend the day walking up and down the halls or talking with one another.[38] Regulations are looser in the hostel, so it functions as a reward for those in the clinic to be transferred there.[39] Surrogates in the hostel have meals prepared by a cook, which, while seemingly luxurious, also allows for control of their diet. They can watch television, and while family members may visit, children are permitted only if the surrogacy process is going smoothly, and husbands are prohibited from staying the night or engaging in sexual activity with their wives for the duration of the pregnancy. Hostel workers control the surrogates' schedule as well, offering activities designed to enhance their skills as what Pande terms "surrogate workers."[40] They might participate in English or computer lessons so that they can communicate with international clients; some surrogates in India do communicate with the intended parents, while others never meet with them. In addition, clinic workers control the birth process itself, scheduling C-sections for a majority of the surrogates, though most of them deliver their own children vaginally.[41] Clinics may also implant as many as five embryos into the surrogate, though the American Society for Reproductive Medicine advises doctors to implant no more than three. In cases where multiple embryos become viable, the clinic may selectively reduce or abort without the permission of the intended parents or surrogate in order to increase the statistical chance of a live birth.[42]

Given these practices, the Indian surrogate may be said to be treated as a machine that manufactures a product, and that product is desirable to consumers because of decreased cost. She is the equivalent of the Asian sweatshop sneaker producer or a South American fruit farmer—unseen by the purchaser, her voice, story, and identity kept secure from the product of her labor. Yet while the sweatshop worker assembles a shoe and the laborer pulls mangos from a tree, the surrogate makes a product interior to herself. Other than the embryo, food, and the medications she takes early in the pregnancy, nothing beside her body is needed for the creation of the new life, and the new life itself develops within and not apart from her. This makes the Indian surrogate's body both producer and the site of production. Yet the practices enacted by doctors and intended parents deny her status as an agent in the producing process. They choose her precisely because of the price point that her body is supposedly worth—a price point lower than her American counterparts—and then seek to limit her agency through practices of control that appeal to intended parents. Doctors and intended parents can treat her as object rather than subject in her role as the site of production. That intended parents may never meet or communicate directly with the surrogate reinforces her status as object.

Intended parents and clinic workers may therefore be said to prioritize the product of surrogacy—the biologically connected baby—above the subjectivity of the surrogate. Phrased differently, personhood and relationship become secondary to the business contract that is designed to produce a more reasonably priced product, which in this case is a baby who shares the genes of at least one parent.

International surrogacy practices in India—at least before the 2017 ban—appeared to reinforce the surrogate as object. That objectivity seems even more dire when one recognizes that India remains a country where individuals with lesser economic means struggle to access basic health care, such that many women cannot afford proper health care for their own children or themselves. However, before the 2017 ban on international surrogacy, their access to care changed during their employment as surrogates, with intended parents providing them access to doctors, medicine, and medical procedures. The surrogates therefore received greater care during employment: they received care beyond what they could afford for their own children only when producing children for wealthier couples.[43] Their bodies, then, had value as a vehicle for the production of the intended parents' child, and received care because of their service in that role.[44]

The Role of Antinatalism in Indian Surrogacy

Understanding the role of antinatalism—where antinatalism is defined as policies that deter childbirth—in Indian society is imperative to understanding how surrogacy operates within its overarching cultural framework and how the surrogate interprets her own experience. Beginning in the 1970s, the government encouraged sterilization, sometimes even forcing it on citizens, though it now primarily promotes antinatalism using a voluntary two-child policy.[45] Under the policy, the government tries to encourage couples to choose sterilization following the birth of their second child and offers incentives to do so, including recruitment for or promotion in government jobs, insurance benefits, and educational discounts; it couples these with disincentives that include the inability to hold public office.[46] Additionally, the government encourages poorer women to use more permanent birth control mechanisms in order to keep the overall population down. As a result, within Indian society there appears to be, either intentionally or not, a state-sponsored attempt at eugenics whereby those without resources find their reproductive options limited by the government, while those with greater resources might find freedom from it, precisely because they are less affected by the state's policies.[47]

Such policies contrast with reproduction politics in the United States, which currently tacitly promotes high birthrates among low-income citizens by hindering access to birth control or abortion clinics.[48] The government offers few resources after births occur, however, in contrast to its economic neighbors, many of which offer extensive parental leave and childcare policies. Those without prior personal affluence may thus find it difficult to provide for children once they are born or to financially thrive because of the costs of childcare, with the consequence that the presence of children for the lower classes may well keep them as members of the lower class. The United States, therefore, tacitly encourages poorer individuals to reproduce while simultaneously depriving them of the economic imperatives needed post-childbirth, a strategy that contrasts with policies in India that seek to prohibit reproduction among the lower classes because of their economic status. The United States may be an outlier in this regard, as India's reproductive agenda represents something of a global trend. Its antinatalist policies resonate with other countries in the Global South that have sought to limit reproduction—especially among their poorest members—in recent decades. In contrast, the Global North has embarked upon the advance of reproductive technologies designed to enhance the capabilities of those with enough means to afford the procedures. In combination, what emerges is a global trend toward limiting the reproduction of the world's poorest members while enhancing the capabilities of its richest. The development of the Indian surrogacy industry thereby functioned as a symbol of this movement: while the nation at large has one of the highest absolute maternal death rates and only 51 doctors per 100,000 residents, it maintained a robust assisted reproduction industry, with assets in the billions, up until the 2017 ban on commercial surrogacy.[49]

The treatment of surrogates before the 2017 ban presents a picture of women whose participation in surrogacy stemmed from economic need and, prior to their becoming surrogates, whose reproduction was considered "wasteful" by societal policies and discourses. The children they produced for intended parents had perceived value beyond that of their own children.[50] However, Pande documents that the women who participated in Indian surrogacy often saw their pregnancies and births as opportunities to transform their identity from wasteful reproducers to "productive" ones.[51] The surrogates Pande interviewed seemed well aware of the contrast between how society viewed their bodies in terms of the creation of their own children and how their bodies could be reinterpreted in their surrogate roles; they also viewed their time in the clinic as an opportunity to strengthen their education—as the clinic offered several such opportunities—or to escape unhealthy or abusive home environments. In this way, the perspective of the Indian surrogate might have differed from those who did not share her context such that, to the outsider, while Indian surrogacy might have seemed de facto exploitive, its ban fully justified, Pande summarizes it thus:

> The negotiations and resistances of these women need to be seen in light of the history of development of biomedicine in India. . . . The surrogates at Armaan are exerting control over their own bodies and lives by using their bodies for labor. The embodied labor performed by the surrogates subverts antinatalist state propaganda and hegemonic narratives that frame the reproductive bodies of poor women as wasteful. At the risk of undermining the power of these subversive narratives, however, I urge readers to notice the unintended consequences of these resistances at the discursive and individual levels.[52]

Israeli Surrogacy

Israeli surrogacy practices initially appear similar to American and Indian ones in that surrogates have lower income than intended mothers, receive compensation for their services, and embark upon a signed contractual agreement with the intended parents. However, its practices are also distinct in many ways. First, Israel's small size makes physical contact between surrogates and parents easier to arrange than in larger countries, so while it is not uncommon for Indian surrogates never to meet their intended mothers and for participants in the United States to have scripted contact, Israeli surrogates often develop close relationships with their intended parents, especially the intended mothers.[53] It is not unusual, for instance, for intended parents to visit often and to accompany the surrogate through all parts of the process, from the embryo transfer to delivery.[54]

In addition, while intended parents frequently have more education and a higher income than surrogates, there tends to be less of an economic disparity between the two parties than there is in the United States or India. In her ethnography of Israeli surrogacy, Elly Teman reports that all surrogates, by law, are unmarried with children of their own. Approximately 30 percent can be considered middle or lower-middle class, meaning that they own cars and homes and hold reliable jobs. They are often able to set the money aside that they receive from surrogacy for future use because they already meet their basic needs through their nonsurrogate employment. An additional 50 percent of women fall into the Israeli lower class, meaning they may hold low-paying jobs and also usually receive government assistance to meet their financial needs. They tend to use the surrogacy remuneration to pay debt or move to a better apartment—in other words, to meet more pressing needs.[55] The final 20 percent are economically impoverished, living in run-down homes and poor neighborhoods and desperately needing the money surrogacy provides.[56] The average surrogate in Israel is less destitute on the whole than the average surrogate in India, while the Israeli average intended parent is correspondingly less wealthy than in the United States. Teman reports that less than 15 percent of intended parents she interviewed could be categorized as wealthy. While many financed their surrogacy procedures, the procedures were still within reach to many in the country, in large part because Israel provides health care as a right of citizenship, so many of the out-of-pocket expenses that intended parents pay in the United States receive coverage through

Israel's universal health insurance policy.[57] As a result, surrogacy is a conceivable option for a couple in the middle class in a way that it is not in the United States.[58] What parents are responsible for financially, then, are those fees that are unrelated to medical procedures themselves, such as the cost of an agency if they use one to find the surrogate or the fee paid to the surrogate in compensation for her time and effort, making their overall out-of-pocket expenses less than they would be in the United States.[59]

That the government supports surrogacy through reimbursement for certain expenses related to it derives at least in part from a pronatalist Israeli ideology. Both Israelis and Palestinians attempt to elevate the role of mothers in order to enhance birthrates and increase the population. The choice not to have children remains socially unacceptable in both cultures.[60] In addition, Judaism's ethics link surrogacy to the perpetuation of the faith, further enhancing the nation's desire to support it.[61] For Judaism to persist, births need to persist, particularly births by Jewish women because it is a woman's genes *and* her gestational ability that confer the faith. The identity of not just the genetic donor but also the carrier thereby becomes critically important in Judaism, with many Orthodox rabbis declaring that a child carried by a non-Jewish woman would itself not be Jewish.[62] Both because of its pronatalist ideology and the Jewish theology surrounding the transmission of religious identity, the Israeli government became heavily involved in regulating surrogacy while also making it more accessible to Jewish residents by applying national health-care funds.[63] This also transformed Israeli surrogacy into a distinctly political event, with government law stipulating that all parties must be of the same religion to participate in surrogacy. It also requires that all intended parents be heterosexual and married and that all surrogates be unmarried and have children of their own. Israel outlaws the use of surrogacy for noncitizens. As a result, no same-sex couples, single individuals, or Muslims have used the government service. Israeli surrogacy essentially functions as a way of perpetuating the Jewish religion, the Israeli state, and the heterosexual family model.[64]

Relationships and Identity Transmission in Israeli Surrogacy

Teman's ethnography describes close relationships between surrogates and intended parents that mutually define the identity of each participant, especially the intended mother and surrogate, who use a variety of praxes and communication patterns to construct their desired identities. While Teman discovers commonalities in the relationships between various participants that she observed during the course of a given pregnancy and in its aftermath, these are not scripted or circumscribed interactions between the surrogate and intended parent as in the American context; rather, these patterns more naturally arise as the relationship between the third party and intended parents develops.

In particular, Teman describes a process she terms the "shifting body," which is enacted through a variety of praxes used by surrogates and intended mothers as they work together to create a family. The shifting body may be broadly defined as the process used by surrogates to distance themselves from the fetuses they carry while simultaneously transferring a maternal identity to the mother; the intended mother, for her part, also adopts praxes that allow her to identify as a mother while simultaneously helping the surrogate to construct her role as hero. Each, then, engages with the other so as to embody the identity she seeks to inhabit.[65]

Surrogates and intended mothers in Israel enact a number of practices that permit this evolving process to occur.[66] A surrogate may refuse to touch her own belly, for instance, instead encouraging the intended mother to touch it because she is the one who must bond with the child.[67] Surrogates may also ask intended mothers to accompany them to ultrasounds or examinations, even requesting that doctors wait until the intended mother arrives to perform them.[68] These moments offer opportunities for the surrogate to help construct the intended mother's future maternal identity and can occur, in part, because the women get to know one another during the pregnancy and birth. The process of the surrogate coconstructing a maternal identity for the intended mother continues in the hospital ward itself. Teman recounts one surrogate who created a ritual to enhance the intended mother's maternal self when she instructed medical staff to place the newborn on the intended mother's belly instead of her own; however, when the birth occurred, and the hospital staff laid the baby on her own belly, the surrogate insisted that they remove the baby because it needed to be with its rightful mother and not with her.[69]

The surrogate thereby capitalizes on normed actions or rituals associated with maternal identity and consciously transfers them to the intended mother in order to establish that woman's maternal self while simultaneously diminishing her own. By distancing herself from the tasks or milestones associated with motherhood—tasks that include touching the pregnant belly or putting the baby on top of the belly postbirth—the surrogate also cultivates a relationship with the intended mother in the process, one built on the exchange of identity between the two women.

While the surrogate coconstructs a maternal identity for the woman who will raise the resulting infant, the intended mother and father seek to construct a hero's identity for the surrogate. Teman explains that this aligns with the surrogate's wishes, as she often sees it as her "mission" to create families for childless couples. This mission, in part, springs from nationalistic loyalty, from a desire to help continue the existence of the nation of Israel by supplying it with citizens. The surrogate thereby becomes a hero by accomplishing the impossible—creating parents out of individuals who could not otherwise have biological children—while also literally assisting with the birth of a relatively new nation.[70] The intended parents help the surrogate begin to live into this heroic identity through gift-giving practices. While some gifts involve the exchange of goods, surrogates tend to prioritize gifts that have a relational component. One surrogate described how important it was to her that the intended mother hugged and kissed her immediately after the baby's birth, tears flowing, before even approaching the newborn.[71] This acknowledgment functioned, to the surrogate, as a gift that reinforced her identity as a hero, as someone who had given a priceless present to the family. Another surrogate mentioned that her intended mother repeatedly expressed appreciation and a commitment to her well-being throughout the pregnancy and after the birth of twins. The surrogate recalled that when she was hospitalized for high blood pressure before to the birth of the newborns, the intended mother's first questions were about who would take care of the surrogate's children. She then went to the store to make sure the surrogate had groceries at home. This same surrogate reported that the intended mother came to doctor's appointments with her and always inquired not just about the well-being of the growing fetuses but also about the well-being of the surrogate. From the surrogate's perspective, this showed a loyalty and commitment to her, and she noticed that continuing after the delivery as well. The surrogate also cited how memorable it was that the intended mother called her the evening they got home from the hospital to make sure she was well, and that on the Sabbath immediately following the homecoming, she insisted that the surrogate come to her house for the circumcision (*brit*) and even waited to perform the ceremony until the surrogate arrived.[72]

Fathers likewise coconstruct the surrogate's heroic identity. One surrogate, for instance, described a powerful conversation with a father who told her, "You are G-d for us," while others referred to the value of gifts offered by fathers as signs of their appreciation.[73] These examples together present a picture of surrogacy in which the surrogate's future self becomes a driving force in her participation in assisted reproduction that other members of the community validate and seek to coconstruct through practices such as gift giving or verbal statements of acknowledgment or appreciation.

While a variety of practices exist at the interpersonal level to help construct the identity of those involved in surrogacy arrangements, the wider Israeli society participates in the construction process as well. The Israeli government requires certain rituals that delineate the identity of intended parents and surrogates, such as a welfare officer who meets with all parties so the surrogate can officially relinquish the child into the custody of the intended parents within forty-eight hours of the birth. Medical personnel also support the delineation of roles in surrogacy relationships.[74] Hospital workers admit surrogates to women's health units while they admit intended mothers to maternity wards, granting intended mothers a bed there and a hospital gown to wear for the remainder of their infants' stays, in addition to an admittance bracelet that gives them access to the nursery. Such practices allow women to inhabit the maternal experience they would have had if they had physically birthed the child.[75]

The aforementioned praxes evidence how members across Israeli society—including doctors, nurses, and government officials—intentionally help both the surrogate and intended mother to construct delineated identities within the reproductive relationship. The women's maternal and heroic identities are thereby built through their relationship, with society at large reinforcing their roles.[76]

Israeli surrogacy affords different import to the role of relationships than the American or Indian contexts do. It is capable of affirming the contributions of all involved parties, empowering both the surrogate and the intended parents in their respective roles so that the experience of surrogacy becomes a transformative moment for each involved party in a positive way. Moreover, the Israeli system allows for the development of relationships between parties, rendering surrogacy an event that is less a business or financial contract than a relational one. Surrogacy therefore becomes predicated upon the acknowledgment of the contributions of all involved parties, mitigating the possibility of exploitation by relationship cultivation, interpersonal acknowledgment, and the empowerment that follows. This is not to say that all Israeli arrangements are ideal or that harm cannot be done, but it is to say that the risks soften, given the supportive structures surrounding participants.[77] In contrast, American and Indian clinics function within the boundaries of societal norms that view surrogacy as a business contract, with the result that participants circumscribe interactions via scripting or anonymity, which creates environments that can reinforce dehumanization or abuse of third parties.

Conclusion

An overview of surrogacy in three different contexts reveals both cultural particularities and some universals. In each culture, the surrogate suffered when intended parents did not acknowledge their relationship to her, either through gift giving or other practices of acknowledgment. Each culture's surrogate also tended to see herself as inhabiting a place of power because her body had the ability to produce what otherwise could not be manufactured: a live baby. However, each culture also used the surrogate to achieve ends that reflected its overarching values, whether that meant perpetuating the biological family or maintaining the birthrate among privileged groups, be it the middle and upper classes in the Indian and American contexts or members of the Jewish faith in the Israeli one. These ethnographic findings in turn have theological import, because the construction of each proposes different understandings of the self as it relates to larger communal units. How to interpret these findings theologically therefore raises questions about what is at stake for the self, the family unit, and the wider community in regard to surrogacy.

3

Hagar, Sarah, and Forms of Socially Constructed Surrogacy

The desire for children is a primal need that extends beyond the individual to the species itself, for the urge to create another human life ensures the survival of the race and the continuation of its particular genetic configuration. Debatably, the reproductive urge is not within control of the individual any more than death is; the body operates as it has been primed to do since life began, to grow from infancy to adulthood, to gather within it the capacity to produce a new generation, and then to fade away, its work done so that the species may endure. Framed this way, it would seem the reproduction is simultaneously an essentialist part of human identity precisely because it is beyond the control of the human being, and yet to reduce reproduction to an urge is also simplistic, because reproduction is inflected by constructs built by culture, values, and politics. In the United States—where the biological family can function as an idol and where "family values" is the phrase that represents all that is moral and good, there exists a quiet assumption that reproduction is a necessary part of adulthood, along with an assumption that it can be controlled. When neither manifests, then the bodies of the infertile become the site where cultural values and the actual capability to embrace them must be negotiated.[1] Such individuals navigate that clash as they marinate in a society that romanticizes children, imaging them as nymph-like creatures who sprinkle crackly, aging adults with the pixie dust of life's meaning. Meanwhile, the desire for the nymph-like creatures paradoxically creates meaning of an unintended variety. Instead of inaugurating hope, optimism, and a sense of legacy or purpose, the desired but not-yet-existing child instantiates a series of potentially traumatic events: months of forcing the body to sexually encounter its partner because an ovulation kit or doctor said it was the best window for conception, medical procedures and surgeries, and repeated failures accompanied by blood that flows for days in either menstruation or miscarriage, signaling that the body cannot be controlled by desire or technology or society's hopes for it. The lack of control, the lack of privacy, and the repeated attempts to create life thus lead to a series of literal or metaphorical deaths, deaths that occur in the name of seeking life and that create a contradictory narrative of society's story line about what parenthood ought to be.

The contemporary adult whose body cannot reproduce finds him- or herself stepping into a timeless human experience in which the body, the self's desires, and society's technological capabilities do not exist in harmony. In this way, the adult who faces infertility or reproductive loss may be said to have less in common with his or her contemporary companions who easily birth families and more shared experience with the biblical matriarch Sarah, whose own suffering emerged from a persistent inability to birth a child of her own coupled with the societal expectation to do so. In Sarah's time even more than today, fecundity was culturally desirable, especially for women, whose place was relegated to the maintenance of the home, whose purpose was primarily to raise children, and whose financial stability depended on her husband and male children. One could surmise, then, that the conflict between Sarah and Hagar might not have emerged had Sarah not operated within the confines of a society that delineated her role so narrowly. She might not have exploited Hagar had she lacked the desire to reproduce or had society not constructed her role as primarily reproductive. What encourages Sarah and contemporary adults to undertake such actions, therefore, may not be not be infertility so much as it is cultural misorientation coupled with limited choices about reproduction. These two preconditions together create an environment in which the mistreatment of others in reproduction can flourish and in which the self of various parties can experience profound forms of alienation.

The Story of Sarah

Sarah, Hagar, and Abraham's reproductive journey is the most developed representation of surrogacy in the Bible, with the story of Hagar's impregnation and the legacy of that pregnancy and birth on her relationship with Sarah and Abraham developed in Genesis 16 and 21.[2] Indeed, the most extensive exploration of the theological implications of surrogacy occurs in the work of Delores Williams, who uses the Sarah and Hagar story to propose a womanist theology that interprets surrogacy as having essentially negative value. The story of Sarah and Hagar works well for Williams' purpose, as Sarah's treatment of Hagar paradigmatically points to the way that surrogacy can become a vehicle for exploitation. In the story, it is Sarah who initiates the surrogacy arrangement when she instructs Abraham in 16:2 to "go in to my slave-girl" so that Sarah "shall obtain children by her."[3] Her statement acts as an explicit performative, one in which her speech generates a new reality as she commands Abraham to engage in intercourse with Hagar for the purpose of conception. In this way, Sarah is the initiator of the reproductive process, her agency exercised through the speech act. While Abraham receives and follows through on the speech act, ensuring its effectiveness, Hagar remains silent until after she gives birth to Ishmael.[4]

The question of why Sarah offers her slave to Abraham is an intriguing one. On the one hand, Sarah takes action to ensure reproduction in a way that accords with her cultural norms: children would have been the expected conclusion to a woman's reproductive story in biblical times, which constructed her role firmly as wife and mother. Indeed, one might argue that the prominence of fertility goddesses in contiguous religions outside of Judaism provide evidence that the ideal woman in the ancient Near East was a procreative woman.[5] The prominence given to maternal identity in turn justified the ability of a mistress who could not reproduce on her own to offer a slave for the task. The slave thereby functioned as a solution to the mistress's inability to enact reproductive agency and provided a way for her to repair what was perceived as a bodily defect because she could use the slave's body as a proxy for her own.

Sarah had further reason to believe that children were supposed to be part of her reproductive story: God promised it. In Genesis 15:4-5—one chapter before Sarah's performative command—God promises Abraham that he will have biological descendants who will be numerous as the stars. As a result, even if one argues that there were limitations to how Sarah could have written an ending to her reproductive story because of the constructed expectations for female identity within her culture, Sarah has an additional reason to believe she would bear children because of the divine promise. As of chapter 16, however, God has not followed through on the reproductive promise made in the prior chapter such that it appears to have misfired. God does not open Sarah's womb, and God's motives for so doing remain elusive.[6] However, fertility remains a good worth having. Sarah, therefore, may not even be presenting Hagar to Abraham because of a perceived defect on her part so much as because of an awareness of her expected maternal identity coupled with an awareness that God does not seem to be keeping the Genesis 15 promise that Abraham would have descendants numerous as the stars. Perhaps Sarah, in rethinking the promise, believed that the mandate for descendants required human initiative. Perhaps she even believed surrogacy could be part of it—after all, God's promise in Genesis 15 is not that Sarah will be biologically connected to the offspring but that Abraham will. Perhaps these justifications motivated Sarah to take matters into her own hands, and perhaps they did not, but regardless, it might be deduced that Sarah believed enough in the importance of paternal identity for Abraham (and likely in maternal identity for herself) that she was willing to go to great lengths to see it manifested. So Sarah executes her reproductive agency with the resources available to her—in this case, the body of Hagar. Hagar thus loses subjectivity—her body, desire, and agency ignored—so that Sarah can write a chapter of her own, and Abraham's, reproductive story.[7]

Sarah's treatment of Hagar is abuse to the eyes of the modern reader—Sarah facilitates a rape, orchestrating a pregnancy Hagar never asks for and presumably does not desire. The modern reader is likely, and should be, appalled by the lengths Sarah goes to, unapologetically, in order to produce an heir for Abraham, including, as Delores Williams summarizes, suffering for Hagar wrought through "slavery, poverty, ethnicity, sexual and economic exploitation, surrogacy, rape, domestic violence, homelessness, motherhood, [and] single-parenting."[8] While Sarah's actions are not excusable, they are at the very least comprehensible when one factors in both the significance of the divine promise and the constructed expectations for her own identity. Societal norms predetermined that her body was meant to be given in marriage and to bear children—or at the very least to raise them, that her desire should be for those children and for her husband, and that her agency should be enacted for the purpose of maintaining their well-being. Her security, in turn, depends on that of her husband and male heirs. It therefore makes sense that Sarah would have taken the course of action that she did, even as one condemns what she chose to do. Her actions might best be summarized by Nelson Mandela's statement, "I am not truly free if I am taking away someone else's freedom, just as surely as I am not free when my freedom is taken from me. The oppressed and the oppressor alike are robbed of their humanity."[9] Sarah took Hagar's freedom by ordering her rape, and in so doing, she compromised something of herself, even if she was not aware of this at the time.

Sarah may well have perceived her reproductive world through a certain lens—namely, that of cultural construction and divine promise—and while one might query whether Sarah would have acted differently were her circumstances different, this is an impossible exercise in biblical extrapolation. What appears more obvious to the reader who observes Sarah's experience of infertility from a distance is that Sarah did not have complete reproductive freedom, and this constriction inaugurated the dilemma of how to embody the reproductive expectations society had for her as well as the divine promise given when she remained unable to conceive. Navigating those expectations did not become any easier following the birth of Ishmael: Sarah never seems to bond with the child, and indeed there is no evidence in the biblical text that she functioned as his mother. Her own maternal relation to Ishmael becomes even more strained following the birth of Isaac, for now both Ishmael and Isaac can claim to be Abraham's heir, as he fathered both children. It is unsurprising, then, that Sarah feels threatened by Hagar and casts her into the wilderness for a second time in Genesis 21, because by that point, Sarah potentially has much to lose: her own maternal identity, her financial legacy, and her spousal identity in relationship to Abraham are all threatened by Hagar and Ishmael.[10] Sarah, in the end, finds herself navigating a complicated set of reproductive relationships that ancient Israelite society structured in a way that seemed designed to pit the infertile woman against the fertile one, so that while Sarah's agency began the reproductive process, her agency could not ensure a simple, happy ending in the face of delicate parental bonds and societal laws.[11]

In this way, Sarah's reproductive struggle shares some commonalities with that of adults—particularly women—in the contemporary United States. While women in the twenty-first-century United States certainly have more options available to them in terms of how they execute adulthood and how they pen their reproductive story, there remains something of a timeless expectation that reproduction will be part of that adulthood, such that refraining from the task remains countercultural.[12] The contemporary woman therefore finds herself asking the same question Sarah must have asked: to what ends will I go to create the child that I am supposed to have? At the same time, the primacy of the biological family does not treat reproductive relationships that involve third parties as the norm, potentially leading to isolation or exploitation of them. As Delores Williams summarizes (with a hauntingly prophetic voice, as she published *Sisters in the Wilderness* before the widespread use of gestational surrogacy):

> Will the law legitimate surrogacy to the point that black women's ovaries are targeted for use by groups more powerful than poor black women? Will surrogacy become such a common practice in wealthy women's experience that laws are established to regulate it—laws that work to the advantage of the wealthy and the disadvantage of the poor? . . . Are American women stepping into an age of reproduction control so rigid that women will be set against each other like Hagar and Sarah? Will the operation of certain reproduction technologies, acting in white women's favor, put even more strain upon the already strained relation between black and white women?[13]

Who Was Hagar?

Some of Hagar's characteristics can be extrapolated clearly from Genesis 16 and 21: she could conceive and bear children; she was Egyptian in origin. Others are not so easy to understand. Her name is itself elusive—in Hebrew, *ha-gar* (הגר) is a noun that translates to "the foreigner," specifically a male foreigner, as the female version of the noun requires an extra suffix at the end (ה) and would be pronounced *ha-gar-ah* (הגרה). While many other names in the Bible derive from Hebrew words or phrases—Sarah's name means "princess," Isaac's means "one who laughs," and Adam's means "man"—Hagar's case is more complicated because as an Egyptian her parents would not have spoken Hebrew, thereby raising the question of why they would have named their child in the language of her future enslavement. Her name, therefore, may well be a signifier for her place within Abraham's tribe, a cloak that displays her role while covering the proper name that identifies her as a unique self.[14]

If Hagar's name resists clarity, her identity in relation to Sarah and Abraham is even more complicated, as she is variously described in

Genesis 16 and 21 as being Sarah's slave (שפחה), Sarah's handmaiden (אמה), and Abraham's wife (אשה). Each descriptor affords Hagar a different degree of autonomy as well as a different degree of legal protection. Ancient legal codes state that Sarah would have had authority over Ishmael if Hagar were a slave, a perspective reinforced by Genesis 16:2, where Sarah suggests that she will be increased through the children birthed by Hagar.[15] As handmaid, however, Hagar would have had more rights, and as wife, she would have more rights and privileges still, though not as many as Sarah had.[16] At stake for Hagar would be the amount of protection she would have received from Abraham, her status in relationship to Sarah, whether she would have been considered Ishmael's mother, and the rights that she and Ishmael would have had within the tribe; as second wife, Hagar and Ishmael may well have been entitled to an inheritance following Abraham's death, provided that Abraham claimed Ishmael as his own child.[17] As slave, however, she would not have been entitled to an inheritance, and she would have been entirely under the control of Sarah, her mistress. As a handmaid/concubine, Hagar would not have received an inheritance but would have had greater privilege within the family—especially in relation to Sarah—than she would have had as a slave.[18]

The conflicting words used to describe Hagar complicate the reader's ability to discern who Hagar was in relation to Sarah and Abraham. It is clear to the modern reader that she is a victim of abuse; it is clear that she was subjected to horrors. However, her conflicting descriptions as slave, handmaid, and wife suggest a lack of clarity about her status in the reproductive narrative and in turn create confusion about Ishmael's status. If Hagar was a slave, then Sarah might have been considered Ishmael's exclusive mother; if a wife, it would have been the reverse. The second casting out of Ishmael and Hagar in Genesis 21 likewise mean different things depending on the invocation of these different terms: as wife, Hagar's expulsion into the wilderness would have involved her losing an inheritance; as a slave, this would not be the case.

While these descriptors create ambiguity around Hagar's rights and privileges, what stands out to the modern reader of this story is the resonance that Hagar's ambiguity has within modern surrogacy discourses and practices. There is no uniform view of or enactment of surrogacy, such that in some cases surrogates find themselves elevated by the process (perhaps most closely mirroring Hagar as wife) and in others they find themselves objectified (most closely mirroring Hagar as slave). Likewise, the abuse of surrogates—such as what has been documented in India—most closely imitates the kind of treatment Hagar would have received in her status as slave, while some of the gifting and identity-constructing measures that Israeli parents undertake could more closely identify the surrogate with the rights afforded to a second wife (though, of course, the modern-day surrogate is not regarded as a wife).[19] Meanwhile, some parents remain skeptical or refrain from surrogacy because they believe that maternal identity is transferred through the process of pregnancy, as opposed to genes. This fear can lead to a desire to remain anonymous from the surrogate or can create tensions between the intended mother and the surrogate in terms of their respective roles in the reproductive process, as imaged by the negative view that Sarah held toward Hagar regardless of whether Hagar is read as slave, handmaid, or wife.

The ambiguity that Hagar's identity receives in Genesis, then, may confuse modern readers, leading them to ask who exactly Hagar is in relation to Sarah and Abraham and Ishmael. But that ambiguity may also be the narrative's experiential strength. In crafting Hagar ambiguously, the biblical text resonates with contemporary experience, mirroring modern practitioners of surrogacy who themselves must figure out whether the surrogate is subject or object, mother or worker, hero or villain in the reproductive narrative.

What Happened to Hagar?

Hagar is an Egyptian woman living with the tribe of Abraham when the reader meets her in Genesis 16. She exists in a subservient position to Sarah in the capacity of slave or handmaid. She has few rights and minimal autonomy. Hagar has no power to object, no position of privilege to invoke when Sarah directs Abraham to impregnate her, and so she is subjected to rape by the patriarch. Whatever desires she had, the reader does not hear of them, as Hagar does not speak in these opening verses of chapter 16, so that her silence reflects the denial of subjectivity Abraham and Sarah impose on her when they violate her agency through rape.[20] Hagar's silence continues after her impregnation; indeed, no one speaks in these early verses except Sarah, who first instructs Abraham to impregnate Hagar and then voices anger after Hagar seems less than pleased with Sarah for her pregnant state of being.[21]

Abraham speaks for the first time in the pericope following Sarah's statement that she blames him for the way that Hagar looks at her, but Abraham does not intervene in the relationship between the two women, instead instructing Sarah to take whatever action she sees fit. Sarah consequently casts Hagar out into the wilderness, where Hagar encounters an angel of the Lord, who advises her to return to Abraham's tribe and to submit to Sarah as her mistress, seeming to make God complicit in Hagar's ongoing abuse. Yet, in these same verses, God also makes two promises to Hagar. The first is that she will have innumerable descendants. This divine mandate offered to Hagar mirrors what God offers to Abraham in chapter 15, elevating her to the level of patriarch with the promise of such a legacy.[22] Second, the angel states that Hagar will have a male child named Ishmael, though the angel does not sugarcoat Ishmael's personality, describing him as "a wild ass of a man, / with his hand against everyone, / and everyone's hand against him; / and he shall live at odds with all his kind" (Gen 16:12). On the one hand, the future offered to Hagar's descendant does not appear rosy—God describes Ishmael in terms that might deflate any parent and names the obstacles he will face in a way that is downright depressing. On the flip side, the promise of a male child ensures a greater degree of protection for Hagar than if she were birthing a girl. A boy potentially could receive Abraham's inheritance; he would have more rights and freedom within Israelite culture. A girl, in contrast, would be nothing but property, in need of a dowry, ultimately destined to leave her mother's side and possibly to repeat Hagar's fate of being raped and abused by others who would always see her as an object that existed for their own gratification and self-advancement. Perhaps, then, within Hagar's societal construction, the promise of a "wild ass of a man" might still be preferable to the promise of a girl.

Genesis 16 concludes with Hagar seeing and naming God, making her the only female in the Bible to so do. Here the reader observes the irony that Hagar receives privilege in the midst of her abuse and indeed receives privilege from God, even as God seems to condone the perpetuation of harm that Hagar experiences at the hands of Abraham and Sarah as she receives directions to return to the home of her abusers. Yet God also seems to have given Hagar what is necessary for her immediate survival, if not for her flourishing: the directions to return to the tribe offer her the material she needs to satisfy what we might call in contemporary parlance the minimum standard of care—food, physical shelter, clothing. And even if they do nothing to promote her flourishing, these resources may be greater than what Hagar could have provided for herself in the wilderness. So Hagar returns to Abraham's tribe, armed not with physical force but with the promise of a future and the immediate prospects for her survival ensured.[23]

Though Hagar goes back to Abraham's fold and remains there until after Ishmael's birth, relationships between Sarah and Hagar do not appear to improve during Hagar's pregnancy, nor does Sarah ever seem to identify as Ishmael's mother. Indeed, Sarah feels so threatened by Ishmael that when the Genesis narrative returns to Hagar's story in chapter 21—after the birth of Sarah's biological son, Isaac—Sarah demands that Abraham exile him and Hagar when she sees the two boys playing together. Depending on Hagar's status as slave, wife, or handmaid, Sarah's response may have been motivated by fear of the economic consequences of Ishmael's birth because ancient Hebrew inheritance laws dictated that a man's firstborn son—not his wife—would receive his financial legacy. This would have been the case if the tribe perceived Hagar as a second wife or possibly as a handmaid, though it would not have applied if she were viewed as Sarah's slave. In other words, in cases such as Sarah's, where a surrogate birthed the firstborn son and the surrogate held a degree of status within the tribe, the resulting child would become the primary inheritor and leader of the family's tribe, according to the right of primogeniture. That would mean increased power for Ishmael and Hagar at the expense of Sarah's status. Were that the case, then both Hagar and Ishmael would have functioned as a threat to Sarah, especially after the birth of Isaac, whom she perceived as the rightful inheritor.[24]

This threat may have led Sarah to demand that Hagar and Ishmael leave her community. On this second occasion, the two depart permanently, this time into the wilderness of Paran, which in the Christian tradition is noted to be a far less hospitable environment than the wilderness setting of Hagar's first departure, which contained a well between Kadesh and Bered.[25] With barely any resources—save a skin of water and some bread—and no one to ask for help, Hagar becomes despondent; not only is she alone in the desert with a child, but she also must procure meals and shelter in a hostile environment, aware that she no longer has the protection of affiliation with a family or house.[26] The overarching family constructions in Hebrew society thus directly affect Hagar's outlook precisely because she is aware of the security provided by familial relationships to individuals who might otherwise be vulnerable on their own. To be part of a family—or a "house"—was not only to share blood ties but also to procure safety. If conflict emerged with outsiders, members of a house would have predetermined physical support, thereby offering them greater protection than they could secure for themselves alone. Slaves who were part of a house also received this protection, meaning that Hagar would have had the security of Abraham's house during her time as Sarah's slave. However, once Sarah and Abraham abandoned her to the second wilderness, Hagar would have found herself without those relationships at the time when she might have needed them most, especially if she encountered hostile nomads or other tribes making their way through the wilderness.[27]

To survive nomadic desert life, then, usually required that one affiliate with a new family; however, this would have been a challenge for Hagar because of her inferior status as an unmarried slave woman, and it may have fallen to Ishmael to negotiate involvement with a new tribe. But there is no definitive evidence that this occurred. Genesis says only that Ishmael dwelled in a wilderness region known as Paran and that Hagar found a wife for Ishmael from Egypt. In this way, Hagar creates a new family, one that will ultimately be led by her son—an Israelite outcast—and his Egyptian wife, who, like Hagar, is a foreigner. From the perspective of the Israelites, this is an unconventional family, to say the least, one led by an "ass of a man" who is the surrogate child of a biblical patriarch but maintains no lasting relationship with that patriarch and whose mother is a foreign slave who found a foreign wife for her son. It is a family that dwells in isolation from other families, building its own tribe in inhospitable environs, without extensive kinship support or access to other familial networks.[28]

In this way Hagar simultaneously experiences challenge and freedom after Sarah casts her out for the second time, because it is in the wilderness that she experiences her deepest despair, and it is also in this wilderness that she discovers an ability to act unencumbered by abuse.[29] Hagar therefore ironically gains agency only when her fertility—the one asset that gave her power in Abraham's tribe—is no longer valuable and indeed would likely have been to her detriment.[30] Her story, then, moves from silence to agency, even as that agency is strangely exercised in the midst of ongoing subjugation and struggle.[31] The story of Hagar, then, lends itself to something of an uncomfortable way of working through theodicy: agency can be procured through victimization.[32] Freedom can emerge, but it emerges through oppression. A slave like Hagar can conquer the odds—thanks to both her own ingenuity and divine solidarity—but at a price. An object can become a subject, but is the journey worth the pain?[33]

On Surrogacy's Inherent Value

The previous chapter's cross-cultural examination of surrogacy revealed a breadth of surrogate experiences. In the United States, the business contract tended to characterize how intended parents related to surrogates, with clinics wielding a fair degree of power in their ability to script the relationships that emerged between parties. In Israel, surrogates and intended mothers often coconstructed one another's roles in a way that addressed the desires of each, while in India, the possibility of harm seemed most evident and the instantiation of harm most clearly documented.

The diversity of surrogate experiences makes any wholesale, essentialist evaluation of modern surrogacy difficult unless one is willing to discard the views of at least some participants. But to do this would be to undermine the wisdom that only they can share: the wisdom of their bodies. Anyone who engages with surrogacy without direct personal experience of it does so in a disembodied way, and yet the body is a necessary component of surrogacy, for no baby is created without the direct contributions of a woman's physical form. To fail to account for this element of the surrogate experience would be to fail to account for the very thing that makes reproduction viable. However, acknowledging the voices of surrogates also means that one must account for the diversity among them, including the ones whose experiences seem to echo Hagar's multilayered account of surrogacy and the ones whose experiences seem more distant from Hagar's experience.

The different accounts of surrogacy seem to suggest that, as in Hagar's account, surrogacy may look very different depending on the constructs that influence the surrogate's experience, the way that the surrogate views the surrogacy itself, and the support she receives from others in the reproductive community. It therefore may be more appropriate to consider three different categories of surrogacy, given current documentations of it, in forms that might be termed constructive, resistive, and injurious.

Constructive Surrogacy Defined

In its constructive manifestation, the locus of surrogacy is one in which agency is free to work in the service of desire, unimpeded by systemic forces and likely supported by them. For example, consider the Israeli surrogate whose doctor respected her desire to wait until the intended mother arrived to perform an ultrasound. The doctor in this example understood that the surrogate, in wanting to distance herself from a maternal role, sought the intended mother's presence in order to firmly establish her own as a hero to this particular family and to manifest her own desire for legacy. Meanwhile, the intended mother appeared for the procedure because she wanted to participate in the identity transfer for her own benefit (her desire for motherhood) and for the benefit of the surrogate, in order to more firmly delineate their respective roles. The example shows the way that a system can uphold self construction when individuals acknowledge the self's desires—in this case, when the medical professionals, intended mother, and surrogate upheld the desires of the latter two participants.

Constructive surrogacy thereby gives the surrogate a chance to exert her agency in a way that emerges from within the culture itself so that the desire she constructs can be sought. It also presents the surrogate as subject rather than object in the surrogacy narrative. In contrast to Hagar—whom Sarah treats as an object, demanding her rape and her subsequent expungement from the tribe—the woman who participates in constructive surrogacy participates as a subject who desires to influence another's reproductive narrative in a particular way, by forming a new life that another will raise.

The question emerges of whether it is possible for a woman organically to name or express desire to participate in surrogacy in this way, especially given the power of social constructs that influence or even determine what it means to be a woman in the Western world. Such constructs often emphasize maternal as well as nurturing or altruistic instincts as "proper" feminine characteristics, so that a woman in the United States is positively reinforced for inhabiting identities of wife and mother and for engaging in self-giving actions and other-directed professions. As a result, the desire to offer children to another reflects both the maternal and the generous self-giving, even self-sacrificial, characteristics that U.S. culture reinforces in women.[34] To offer the body to a pregnancy for a child she will not keep therefore becomes the ultimate act of altruism and, in turn, the ultimate manifestation of the feminine self in the Western world.[35] Thus, the woman who becomes a surrogate for altruistic motives or because she loves children or loves being pregnant not only adheres to but also uplifts what a woman ought to be. In contrast, the surrogate who participates in the procedure for financial reasons might be characterized as self-serving or mercenary.

To the extent that the social construction of a woman's identity influences the decision to be a surrogate, then, her decision cannot be said to be freely desired.

Such an argument holds sway insofar as the reality of social constructs endangers a woman's ability to freely choose to participate in surrogacy. It also renders difficult the ability to discern the difference between actual and stated motives in surrogates because of the role that social constructs may play in the public vocalization of their desires, because the surrogate may well know that it is more socially acceptable to state altruistic and not financial motives. However, what such an argument downplays is the potential that—social constructs aside—humans at their best might *want* to share what they have with others, even in spite of the influence of social constructs, and that such sharing is a profound good. It would be, in other words, a better world if humans freely shared the resources they have for the sake of others who do not have them, and quite a sad world if they did not. Freely expended generosity epitomizes some of the best qualities of humans: the ability to consider the needs of a body beyond one's own, the ability to empathize with the needs of others, and the ability to act in order to make the life of another person better. Theologically, such human-initiated generosity also mirrors the freely offered generosity of a God who shared God's self in creation, in the life of Jesus, and through continued commitment to human flourishing.

It is freedom, however, that becomes pivotal to a positive understanding of generosity. It is, after all, quite a different matter to be coerced—either explicitly, in the case of Hagar, or implicitly, as in the cases where social constructs hold significant power—into sharing what one has for the sake of another. In constructive surrogacy, therefore, freely offered generosity characterizes the surrogate's agency such that the influence of explicit or implicit external powers such as social constructs becomes inconsequential.

One potential vision of constructive surrogacy—though by no means the only one and potentially not immune from social constructs itself—would be the image of the surrogate as ally.[36] As ally, the surrogate would be someone who is freely using the privilege and power that she possesses—in this case, her reproductive privilege—in the service of those who lack it, motivated by faith, hope, and love: faith in the reproductive story that the individual or individuals who cannot reproduce seek to enact; hope that as a surrogate she can help; and love for self and other as the root of a relationship, where love is defined as desiring what is best for the person in question. Aside from these three theological virtues, the surrogate may also be aided by the four cardinal virtues of prudence (here defined as the ability to discern what it means to construct the self and the selves of others); justice (here defined as the desire to exert agency to manifest what is right in regard to self construction as opposed to what is the societal norm or privileged); fortitude (here defined as the strength to do what seems right when it comes to self construction as opposed to what is the societal norm or privileged); and temperance (here defined as the ability to know when self construction involves restraint or saying no).[37] Constructive surrogacy, therefore, is not demanding that a given woman with reproductive capabilities use those abilities to help others reproduce, nor is it suggesting that all individuals who face reproductive difficulties ought to turn to a surrogate. Rather, constructive surrogacy predicates itself upon careful discernment, undertaken in community, that seeks to disrupt the power of social constructs for both the intended parents and the surrogate so that each can make beneficial reproductive decisions to write their reproductive stories in a way that upholds the three components of the self.

Resistive Surrogacy

The surrogate is still able to exert agency in resistive surrogacy; however, the context in which that exertion occurs is different from that of constructive surrogacy. Where the surrogate operates in a system that provides systemic support for authentic self construction in constructive surrogacy, she operates in a system that does not provide much, if any, systemic support in resistive surrogacy, or the social constructs of the system do not freely permit the exercise of desire and agency on the part of the surrogate. A number of the Indian surrogates described in the prior chapter fit into this category. These women found themselves enmeshed in a society that sought to control their fertility and feminine identity. The clinic they worked with did little to support them, curtailing their ability to exercise, dictating their meals and what visitors they could see, and scheduling C-sections and selective reductions without their consent. The women who participated in surrogacy under these conditions appear to have experienced enormous quantifiable violations, yet they also found ways to exert agency in order to resist total subordination. In this way, they refrained from participating in their own objectification but instead found creative ways to function as subjects and construct the self despite external obstacles. For example: surrogates in India enacted their own agency by successfully advocating for a vaginal delivery with doctors, thereby achieving the root desire for control over their bodies, or by using their time in the hostel to further their education, gain skills they could use in the workforce following their delivery, or escape from an unhealthy home environment.[38] They also constructed a surrogacy narrative that imaged themselves as empowered producers, as women who were able to achieve what the men in their lives could not—a degree of financial stability. This perspective allowed the women to elevate their bodies above the dominant Indian cultural view of them—namely, that the bodies of women who participate in surrogacy are taboo because they represent a form of body selling akin to prostitution—and reclaim them as a site of positive productivity.[39] They also acted to reframe their own reproductive value; whereas their ability to reproduce external to surrogacy only increased their poverty, leaving them with more mouths to feed, more education to provide for, or more dowries to grow, they used their reproductive capability through surrogacy to achieve greater financial and social freedom.[40] These women might be most likened to Hagar the second wife (אשה) or Hagar the handmaid (אמה), because like Hagar, they found a way to survive in the wilderness or within a social structure that sought to subordinate them. However, the culture at large offered them little power and did not value them as agents, so that they had to find creative ways to exercise agency, to cultivate a self, while being marinated in a system designed to eradicate it. In other words, these surrogates were not Sarah—who might be said to epitomize female privilege while still holding the subordinate cultural position of female—or Abraham, who held a dominant cultural position thanks both to his gender and his role in the tribe. Indian surrogates attained neither of these privileged social loci; however, to say that they had no privilege by virtue of their complete inability to exert agency would also be reductive.

The steps that Hagar or Indian surrogates took to exercise their agency in this context might be labeled acts of resistance.[41] The successful acts of resistance undertaken by Indian surrogates do not necessarily facilitate an unmitigatedly positive outcome; because the surrogate continues to act within a system designed to subvert her own agency, even as she finds ways to exert her self, she does so within a societal structure that actively facilitates reproduction for powerful individuals while thwarting it for those who lack power or privilege, including her.[42] This type of resistance signifies what Catherine Keller refers to as the "productive ambivalence of postcolonial theory," or the idea that "possibility opens within oppression."[43] Therein lies the irony: an Indian woman may experience significant quality-of-life improvement following her surrogacy experience, just as Hagar may have been better off at the end of her life as the matriarch of a new—if isolated—family unit that Ishmael and his Egyptian wife helped create. Yet these positive increases in status or freedom or finances appear significant only in relation to the women's past, and even so, one wonders whether they amount to enough. For most Indian women, the amount of money they received helped, but it did not significantly improve their ability to provide for themselves or to manifest the dreams they had for the children—despite promises that receiving what amounts to five years of their income would transform their social location—and many returned to homes that lacked supportive husbands or extended family. Likewise, Hagar lived out her final days in the wilderness, mother to a son who, according to the angel of the Lord, is not exactly easy to like or full of social graces. Thus, possibility did indeed open up for these women thanks to their resistive capabilities, but perhaps the resistance they expressed facilitated their survival more than it facilitated their ultimate freedom from oppression. Still, while liberation might be ideal, survival is significant.[44]

Resistive surrogacy is therefore simultaneously a site of oppression and an opportunity for subverting it. It is ambiguous, even as it is full of potential, its hope lying in the reality that resistance is possible even when the overarching system is designed to thwart it. It is like a door, slightly ajar, that leads from a darkened room to a lit one. A person may catch a glimmer of light from the darker space, but what one sees is merely a slice of the fullness of the room itself. The glimmers of resistance that historic and contemporary surrogates offer function in much the same way, presenting glimpses of what more permanent systemic change could look like were the circumstances different.

Injurious Surrogacy

What separates resistive from injurious surrogacy is precisely that glimpse. While resistive forms still allow the surrogate to exert agency, injurious surrogacy does not. It traps the surrogate so that she has no ability to act on behalf of her own desires and no opportunity to pursue her basic needs. She is rendered fully an object, her self disregarded by those with the power to do so.[45] The surrogate functions as Hagar did as slave (שפחה), having no rights, no privilege, no power. To that end, the portion of Hagar's surrogacy experience surrounding her forced impregnation might be said to emblematize injurious surrogacy, because by raping her Abraham disregards her root desire for bodily integrity and any attempts at agency she may have made to secure it. Sarah is no less culpable because by ordering her rape she actively participates in Hagar's objectification, caring no more for Hagar's desire for bodily integrity than her husband does. Likewise, in contemporary surrogacy, those with power—doctors, intended parents—can regard the surrogate as object in such a way that the harm they inflict on the surrogate's self has the possibility of remaining unredeemed unless something in the system shifts.[46] The freedom and generosity that characterize constructive surrogacy are therefore absent, and the resistance that hallmarks resistive surrogacy is nowhere to be found. In this final form, the surrogate is Hagar in the wilderness of Paran: helpless, weeping, unable to act.

The difference between injurious and resistive or constructive surrogacy is therefore not determined by the act of surrogacy itself, because if meaning rested within the act, then that meaning could apply across contexts. Rather, surrogacy's meaning emerges through the way that participants exhibit faith, hope, and love toward each other and through the way that the overarching cultural values of the system affect their ability to do this. As a result, surrogacy looks very different in different times and places because of cultural influence: surrogacy is not the same in Israel as it is in India or the United States or in the experience of the Hagar. Nor is it the same within each individual surrogate unit of intended parents, doctors, and surrogate in any given context, because these individuals exist within different microsystems of values and constructs, influenced by individual experiences that cause them to have unique understandings of their own selves, their own role in the surrogacy process, and their own sense of agential strength. As a result, external forces shape their understanding of their bodies, their desires, and their sense of agency, and ultimately this affects the meaning they ascribe to surrogacy itself and the possibility that injurious surrogacy will manifest.

4

The Self, Corporate Sin, and Cultural Misorientation

Categorizing forms of surrogacy reinforces the fact that surrogacy's value rests largely on its context, its execution, and the extent to which participants validate the three self components. Constructive surrogacy works best in contexts where all participants have relationships with one another that respect the full self of the other, including the other's agency, and where freedom and generosity can coexist, unencumbered by external forces. Injurious surrogacy is most likely to appear in systems with skewed power dynamics where the "haves" need not validate the agency of the "have-nots." Constructive surrogacy can thus rapidly transform to injurious surrogacy. In the American context, for instance, injurious surrogacy may occur if parents press a surrogate to selectively abort when she had clearly stated previously that she would not, or if they never acknowledge her presence in the reproductive process.[1] In both these scenarios, the intended parents act in ways that harm the surrogate, but it would be reductive to say they undertake these behaviors in isolation from the cultural system in which they operate. Parents cannot order a selective reduction, for instance, without a doctor who is willing to perform it or laws that permit it or an agency that constructs the surrogate contract in a way that would allow it. The execution of the parents' decision, therefore, is not successful because of their wishes alone. Their ability to inflict injury on the surrogate results from the tacit compliance of other members of the culture who validate the intended parents' desires as more authoritative than the surrogate's.

Having said all that, the surrogate is not the only one who can be negatively affected in the surrogacy process: constructive surrogacy could likewise become injurious if a doctor sat down with a couple, after years of stalled attempts at conception and miscarriages, with photos of live babies and cards from grateful parents on the desk, and handed them a bulletin about surrogacy and told them that this was their only remaining hope to have a family.[2] That doctor impinges on the agency of the couple because, speaking from a place of power, she tells the couple how to proceed rather than engaging in an open conversation about the many options they actually have and how they themselves prefer to end their reproductive story. Again, in this scenario, the doctor is not acting in isolation but rather is representing the overarching beliefs of the culture in which she operates, namely the belief that the biological family is superior to other forms of family and the belief that her role as a doctor is to facilitate the live birth of a baby and not to facilitate the overall health of a family unit. Intended parents may therefore find themselves inclined to participate in surrogacy without fully considering other ways to narrate their reproductive story because of the power accorded to their physician and the culturally normed beliefs that the physician represents and for which he or she advocates.

These illustrations reinforce that reproductive choices occur within the confines of a system so that individual reproductive decisions represent the execution of that system's values and beliefs. Reproduction, then, is not a private matter. It may be discussed quietly between individuals, and actions may be taken to facilitate it in the privacy of one's bedroom; however, dominant cultural values hold great power to influence an individual's reproductive agency. It therefore becomes difficult to hold the individual accountable for something like injurious surrogacy without reference to the collective whole because societal politics and priorities affect the individual's outlook and potential actions.

Surrogacy's Relationship to Corporate Sin as Cultural Misorientation

Consider the biblical Sarah again: while Sarah's social reality differs substantially from that of the modern parent in the United States or other parts of the Western world—she would not have known, for instance, about women's genetic connection to their offspring, what Sarah shares with contemporary men and women who cannot bear children is the pressure to do so. Contemporary adults spend vast quantities of money and exert incalculable emotional energy so that their bodies will perform the task of reproduction and simultaneously maintain their biological lineage. Not unlike Sarah, they are willing to go to great lengths to achieve this end. They inject themselves with hormones, take ultrasounds of their ovaries, harvest their eggs, freeze their embryos, and implant them into the wombs of other women because it creates the child they desire the most. They do all within their power to end the reproductive story so that their genetic material survives, since that is what appears to be the best way forward.

The web of forces that maintains the privilege afforded biological reproduction over other forms of family creation may be considered a kind of cultural misorientation, or, in theological language, a form of sin. Sin here is not defined by a transmission of original guilt through sexual intercourse at conception but rather by the reality that humans emerge into a broken world that they must navigate, and in so navigating they inevitably become both victim and perpetuator of its broken practices.[3] The cultural systems that perpetuate a collective misorientation in matters of reproduction, therefore, do not originate within the individual. They encompass assumptions about the idealization of youth over age, generally negative views of childless living, linguistic discourses that structure and in turn provide power to certain connotations of "family," and the patriarchal desire to perpetuate one's genes to the point that perpetuation becomes a form of idolatry. They are insidious, hidden, enmeshed with a complex set of beliefs and practices ranging from economic ones that make adoption financially inaccessible to a variety of prejudices against children who need to be adopted, especially children in the foster system who often are at an intersectional disadvantage because of physical or psychological differences, developmental delays, skin color, economic background, or age. Such ideologies collude and combine to act as a form of cultural, corporate sin that, regardless of its origins, keeps people from freely realizing their identities as fully formed children of God, a state of sin that remains, regardless of adult reproductive capability, a state that endures in children, regardless of whether they are created via a surrogacy procedure that cost $120,000 or via biological reproduction to parents who were incapable of raising them such that they became wards of the state. These beliefs wield power over all participants in surrogacy—over intended parents who must try to make the best possible choices in a culture that is not arranged for them to do so, in some cases causing them to instantiate further harm even when that is not the goal; over surrogates who must navigate a system that privileges those with economic means as well as constructs of feminine identity and the biological family; and over children birthed through the procedure.

Cultural Misorientation and the Intended Parent

Acknowledging the role of cultural misorientation changes the contours of what is at stake for intended parents in a theological discussion of surrogacy. It acknowledges the role of external beliefs that affect choice, and it acknowledges the limits placed on their own freedom. The impact of this lack of freedom cannot be overstated and may initially appear surprising. Many individuals who turn to surrogacy today come from places of privilege, be they economic, racial, educational, or a combination of the three. They might be said to be the equivalent of tribal leaders in ancient times, and in this way they encounter surrogacy from the same social location that Sarah and Abraham did millennia ago, for they hold a certain degree of power that allows them to counter the stigma of childlessness and to accept the value placed on biological children within society through their employment of the surrogate.

And yet, even for those who hold these privileged locations in society, cultural assumptions about the ideal family place them at a disadvantage because they cannot inhabit what is considered the familial norm. In regard to reproduction, they lack the privilege they enjoy elsewhere in their lives because of the way that American culture perceives the importance of fertility. Awareness of that social location may play a significant role in their choices, even going so far as to determine their reproductive desires.[4] Cultural misorientation can therefore affect what intended parents believe about reproduction generally, how they understand their own experiences of reproduction, and how they choose to act in light of their own reproductive difficulties, in turn transforming what might be a root desire into a negative projected one.

Cultural misorientation may also affect the processing of reproductive trauma. As intended parents navigate this trauma, they may be cognitively saturated by the limits of society's own understanding of how to formulate the family. Their ability to write an ending to their reproductive story freely, therefore, is impinged, despite it being the key to their own healing. Summarily, the contemporary American adult view of reproduction is potentially as clear as the view obtained through sunglasses: there is a coloring to it that tints reality with a given light. But unlike individual sunglasses, it's difficult to remove the collective ones when society—consciously or unconsciously—perpetuates philosophies and enacts policies that keep them on. The individual adult's projected desires thereby develop under the influence of these culturally misoriented sunglasses, and the agency they exert in turn bears their tint.

If cultural misorientation affects intended parents such that they make their reproductive decisions while embedded in a system that misses the mark, then the question of whether intended parents can surmount the system arises.[5] Put in theological language, the issue becomes whether personal redemption can emerge when an individual is stuck in a location of corporate sin. This is not the same as asking whether there can be redemption for parents who experienced infertility or reproductive loss (such phenomena are the by-products of bodily vulnerability, not of sin itself). Neither is it the same as asking whether an individual is responsible for the sin of the whole because a single person may act from within the whole or contribute to it, but the corporate system still exists beyond individual scope. Nor is it the same as asking whether the individual should solve the cultural misorientation of the whole. If a group collectively contributes to the problem, then the group must collectively contribute to its solution: it makes as much sense for an individual to solve the problem of collective cultural misorientation as it does for a single bee to deconstruct a beehive that tens of thousands of its companions arranged while the other bees lie around and snack on leftover honey. The issue is therefore not what it looks like for corporate sin to be individually redeemed but what it looks like for corporate sin to be corporately redeemed.

It therefore makes sense to have a greater awareness of how cultural misorientation affects the individual. As explicated in earlier chapters, reproductive trauma often affects the self, with particular relevance to the enactment of agency. What follows, then, is an analysis of how cultural orientation affects the agency of all parties involved in surrogacy procedures.

Agency and the Intended Parent

Cultural misorientation may be the overarching framework in which intended parents operate such that they process infertility and reproductive loss through its lens. In other words, infertility and reproductive loss are stressful, upsetting, and potentially traumatic events in any context, but cultural misorientation may exacerbate how a person is able to respond to these events because of the way that it encourages individuals to understand the self and the primacy afforded to the biological family as a good worth having in adulthood. When one cannot access what is privileged, suffering emerges in a way that it would not if the good were not valued or idolized.[6]

Misorientation also informs how intended parents might navigate the agential constraint that accompanies the aftermath of infertility and reproductive loss, shaping their experience of the options available as they seek to restore agency. As a result, their moral framing, their understanding of their own social acceptability and the financial reality of their reproductive options may all be affected by cultural misorientation, constraining their choices as they craft a new ending to their reproductive story.[7]

Finally, cultural misorientation also leads to suffering in cases of infertility and reproductive loss because of the potential it has to alienate individuals from relationships that are pivotal to their reproductive story. That alienation may affect parents, surrogates, and children through three forms: self-alienation, community alienation, and divine–human alienation.

Form One: Self-Alienation and the Intended Parent

Cultural misorientation does not address the kind of grief that occurs in the aftermath of the eradication of expectations and dreams, both of which can be understood as needs that extend from the root desires for stability, relationship, and self-actualization. In the case of intended parents, the inability to biologically reproduce when one desires to do so is not so much a problem related to the status of the body as it is a problem related to the ability to exert agency in the first place, given that agency is a primary component of the self. Being unable to act thereby transforms the self from subject to object, and it is that status as object that in turn stultifies personhood.[8] Individuals therefore do what they can to reconstitute subjectivity because, being alienated from the self, they seek to find it again. As a result, the theological frame through which to discuss intended parents' experiences is not so much sin or theodicy as it is theological anthropology.

Self-alienation becomes pivotal to thinking theologically about intended parents: The inability to enact reproduction can be blindsiding for those whose hoped for reproductive story included the presence of biological children, causing them to feel alienated from the identity they constructed for themselves and from their own assumptions about what it means to be a creative being. However, these intentions may also be determined by cultural constructs that emphasize the self as a physically reproductive creature above the self as a child of God. To that end, part of self-alienation may stem from assumptions about what constitutes the foremost grounding of the self's three components, that the accidents (to invoke Aristotle) of the body or its instrumental capabilities ground the self more than self's intrinsic nature of possessing dignity because all humans are made in God's image.[9]

The kind of redemption that the intended parent seeks is therefore not redemption from sin but rather redemption of identity. This translates in practice to the process of individuals reconstituting who they are in light of reproductive events, with the guiding question being one of agency: how is one to exert agency as a subject when the conditions in which one exists seem to be trying to take it away? Asking this question opens the possibility for redeemed personhood, allowing individuals to discover how to exert themselves as creative beings in spite of unforeseen circumstances.[10]

Form Two: Community Alienation and Intended Parents

The alienation intended parents experience is not entirely about the individual being separated from his or her own sense of self. It is also a sense of alienation from the children with whom that individual sought relationship. Individuals who dreamed of biological children established relationships with the potential of those humans, and grief emerges with the death of that potential. This causes intended parents to become separated from relationships they hoped would be part of their lives.

Alienation from others—in this case, potential children—ties back to the essence of personal agency as simultaneously independent and relational.[11] As agent, a person not only makes an independent decision to act but also decides with whom to act. The elementary school child who decides she wants to play tag decides both that she, as an individual, wants to play the game but also that, in order to play the game, she has to engage with others on her team and the opposing team. In deciding to play tag, therefore, the girl is both deciding what she wants to independently do while also deciding that she wants to do it with others, likely specific others.

A person who cannot exert agency to either act independently or to be in relationship therefore feels not only self-alienation but also alienation from the community, just as the child who wants to play tag but who cannot find anyone in her neighborhood to join her will likely feel. In the case of intended parents, then, the inability to enact their own reproductive story is also an alienation from sought-after relationships with children entrusted to their care. The second phase of redemption for intended parents, then, is the restoration of those sought-after relationships.

Intended parents will ideally have the opportunity to resolve relational agency by reconstructing their reproductive stories in a way that allows them to continue to exercise relationality. The trouble, however, is that cultural misorientation can affect this process. Individuals exist in a pressurized system that sets an implicit hierarchy for familial relationships, with biological relationships ranking ahead of other forms. Yet being told that there is one right way to act—whether that message is implicit or explicit—when one is having difficulty acting at all becomes another type of objectification because it takes away individual choice. This is how cultural misorientation affects intended parents: it affects the perception of which choices are available for relationship cultivation and how viable they are.

In contrast, chapter 1 noted that healing from infertility and reproductive loss is most effective with the use of nondirective methods that offer individuals the possibility to end their reproductive story in a number of ways. This means that individuals may determine that the relationships they seek are ones with adopted children or foster children, that they desire a relationship not only with a child that they will raise but also with gamete donors or surrogates, or that they prefer to practice nurturing relationships in ways that are not related to traditional forms of parenthood. Pivotal here is that the outcome is secondary to the process of ending the sense of alienation from others. In other words, the possibility for restored subjectivity emerges because it becomes possible for the individual to write an ending to the reproductive story that misorientation does not encumber. But for this process to become a reality, cultural beliefs and structures need to be expanded so that all choices become equally available and desirable. This involves a collective reorientation of human life such that certain children are not seen as having value over others due to their genetic makeup, skin color, financial background, intellectual abilities, age, or the history of the adults who provided their DNA. It also involves societally implementing structures that support parents of children who do not fit the norm of what an American child should be, including children with unique physical, psychological, or cognitive traits, children of different racial backgrounds or who come from different countries, and children who are adopted at an older age. It involves, in short, the entire culture becoming more intentionally committed to the belief that all children have equal dignity, leading in turn to actions and policies tailored to meet these children's unique needs and the needs of the parents who commit to loving and raising them. Such a shift in cultural beliefs and actions would lead to an environment in which individuals with reproductive difficulties could more freely exert agency as they discerned what parenthood means for them.

At the individual level, therapists, religious professionals, spouses, friends, and medical professionals can help an individual recover lost subjectivity because of the way that they, within their roles or fields of expertise, provide the individual with opportunities for personal meaning-making. They are in privileged positions to help the individual write a new reproductive story—a story still premised in the same root desire but expressed in different projected ones—and then discover what it means to both independently and relationally enact it. It is therefore the job of such experts to become aware of, name, and press against cultural misorientation so that the intended parent discovers a sense of self that is free from its influence.

Finally, terminating autonomous views of parenthood is essential to terminating community alienation, a challenge because the privilege afforded the nuclear family in the United States could be considered a case study in the illusion of parental autonomy: the ideal American street contains single-family houses, perhaps in walking distance to a school or store. The ideal American parents do not live with their in-laws, adult siblings, or grandparents. They can provide independently for the financial needs of their children and have time to prepare meals for them, chauffeur them to school and activities, and throw them birthday parties. They do not share cars or financial resources with their neighbors but rather see the plot of land on which they live as their domain, the one place on Earth over which they have control. Reproduction therefore becomes part of the culturally privileged narrative that the ideal American family functions independently. Yet this too is a form of misorientation—as well as a falsehood—because communal relationships are essential to both daily living and to reproduction: the schools that parents drive American children to are funded collectively by taxpayers; the cars they use to make the drop-off are hammered and drilled by a set of anonymous workers; the child learns her ABC's thanks to a teacher who uses worksheets provided by an education consultant and printed on paper harvested by workers paid the minimum wage to cut down trees. Known and unknown humans therefore participate to allow the American nuclear family to maintain the illusion of independence, when even this brief analysis indicates that the simple act of attending elementary school could not occur without collective assistance. Americans may therefore imagine themselves to be independent beings, yet they rely on itinerant farm workers to harvest their produce, carpenters to craft their dining room tables, factory workers to sew their clothes and sneakers, chemists to balance their water supply, and engineers to design the cars that take them to work.

The illusion of the autonomous nuclear family therefore mirrors the reproductive autonomous illusion. As with the daily life of the family, in the sphere of reproduction, the sperm needs an egg; the resulting embryo needs a womb; the womb needs food harvested by a farmer to help the embryo grow; the woman who provides the womb needs medical, physical, and emotional support; and in the end the baby needs individuals beyond its parents in order to survive. For children to grow and thrive, they necessarily enter into a network of relationships with grandparents, aunts, uncles, cousins, siblings, teachers, coaches, friends, other parents, activity directors, and bus drivers who all contribute to the well-being of the child.[12] The parent may be responsible for overseeing the salutariness of these relationships, but the parent alone cannot provide for all these needs any more than a given adult can exist in isolation. Parenthood, then, requires that one become part of the "village" that it takes to raise the child, which in turn means that relationships including and beyond the one sought with offspring are the ultimate good that emerges from reproduction. Denial of this becomes one more manifestation of cultural misorientation that needs to be collectively named and addressed.

Reflection on current surrogacy practices reinforce this assertion: constructive models of surrogacy place relationships between parent(s) and surrogate at the foreground such that all participants thrive because they carefully cultivate relationships that make each individual's desires heard and that support each other's agency. In so doing, each allows the self of the other to flourish. Injurious surrogacy, in contrast, functions as a breeding ground for exploitation when participants fail to recognize the value of their relationships; it renders Hagar a slave and makes intended parents into modern versions of Sarah and Abraham. Examples include scenarios where parents treat the surrogate as a gene carrier as opposed to a subject, situations where the surrogate objectifies the parents by using her own fertility as way to exert power over them, and arrangements where all parties remain anonymous or where parents do not tell the child of the surrogate's involvement in the pregnancy.[13] Such situations illustrate the fact that the constrained agency—and resulting suffering and alienation—of intended parents can be contagious, can transmute into similarly constrained experiences for surrogates. Moreover, the cultural emphasis on genes further aggravates the possibility for exploitation. The cultural pressure to reproduce can drive intended parents to undertake actions that inflict harm on another, harm they may be aware of or harm of which they may be ignorant. The irony, however, is that the surrogate is chosen precisely because intended parents are trying to make good on their suffering—trying to write endings to their reproductive story that give it meaning and that make sense of what appears to them to be an existential surd—and not because they seek to harm another woman.[14] This becomes the tragedy of cultural misorientation, that in seeking to resolve suffering and restore agency, parents may further perpetuate it, inflicting agential constraints on another in the name of a child who can justify the suffering that infertility or reproductive loss instantiated in their lives.

Form Three: Divine–Human Alienation and Intended Parents

Infertility and reproductive loss can cause individuals to feel alienated from God, and they may question whether their inability to bear children emerged as a form of divine punishment for defective character or a judgment of their ability to parent, despite the compelling argument that God does not use utilitarianism to evaluate human beings but rather upholds human beings and loves them simply because of their existence. However, in their quest for meaning, humans may not necessarily interpret reproductive loss or infertility this way. Instead, they may interpret it through the lens of what Marilyn McCord Adams calls a "horrendous evil"—namely, the kind of event that makes one question the positive meaning of life.[15] While Adams never describes infertility or reproductive loss in this way, her description of horrendous evils as events that instantiate existential questioning about the overall good that God delivers to a single human life resonates with the experiences of intended parents who feel so derailed by the inability to carry out their dreams that they question the entire purpose of their premortem existence.

Adams proposes that God responds to horrendous evils by making the life of the individual good on the whole, but for this to happen, humans must want to be part of a divine–human relationship that rightly orders itself as friendship, if not in premortem existence then postmortem. This is not the kind of friendship where two parties come together and blithely gossip, go to the mall, or play a game of basketball. In contrast, they enter into "mature friendship" with God and seek to engage in an act of meaning-transformation alongside the divine.[16]

Adams' image of divine–human friendship as a way to facilitate the defeat of evil through the process of meaning-making resonates with the psychological findings on reproductive trauma that suggest healing emerges when individuals are given the freedom to construct meaning from loss and write an ending to their reproductive story that derives from that meaning. Theologically, then, what emerges is that meaning-making requires relationship, such that alienation from the divine contributes to the perpetuation of suffering.[17] It also emerges that there is value to authenticity within the divine–human relationship, value for both God and humans to be acknowledged for who they are and what they can contribute to restitution. Alienation from God therefore takes form when intended parents project motivations onto God for reproductive loss and infertility that counter God's desire for friendship with creation, and when they assume that God evaluates individuals by what they can do rather than what they are. Redemption occurs through the process of accepting that infertility and reproductive loss do not emerge from personal fault or defect but rather arise from the material vulnerability that is an inherent part of material creation.[18] It also involves a personal willingness to be open to the possibility that divine intimacy emerges when one ceases to project either motivation or outcome onto God but rather experiences how God acts in the world qua God as friend.[19] By way of biblical example, just as the disciples on the road to Emmaus could not recognize Jesus for who he was when they felt certain he was just another human stranger en route from one location to another, so contemporary humans find themselves alienated from God when they allow cultural misorientations to guide their narrative about how God works rather than allowing God alone to do that work. Hence, when they believe that God can redeem their experiences only by forming them as biologically grounded parents, they miss an opportunity to cultivate a relationship with God, rooted in friendship, that offers creative possibilities for meaning-making and subsequent healing.

Form One:
Self-Alienation and the Surrogate

Paul writes in his First Letter to the Corinthians that each human receives unique gifts from the Spirit, or in theological language, charisms, and it becomes the calling of the Christian community to discover and uphold the diversity of gifts that God instills in creation. A Christian might wonder how to interpret surrogacy in light of this text, as the surrogate's commitment to using her body to create new life for others to raise can simultaneously be read as a charism and as an exploitive act. The roles of desire and agency distinguish one from the other, because as a woman exercising her unique charism, the surrogate participates out of a sense of personal desire and chooses to undertake the risks of pregnancy and birth, whereas desire and agency are overlooked in cases where others exploit her reproductive ability.[20]

It is perhaps impossible to draw a firm conclusion about what surrogacy can be for the surrogate outside of reference to how a given culture affects its practice. In the United States, surrogates often operate within a business contract with clearly drawn boundaries and limits, perhaps reflective of the emphasis the culture places on capitalism and independence. In India, surrogates usually come from great destitution, destitution that emerges from the country's legacy of the caste system and colonialism. In Israel, the surrogate's contributions are valued in part because of the country's religious beliefs. In each, the country's reproductive policies and overarching discourses concerning maternal identity influence the practice of surrogacy. The impact of culture becomes so crucial to understanding the surrogate's experience that systemic influences are a necessary part of discussions of it.

To consider surrogate self-alienation is therefore to consider the impact of constructs and discourses that affect the individual. Self-alienation can occur for the surrogate when she is unable to make choices based on what most fully allows her to embody the charisms that reflect who she is, because the charisms of one woman are not the charisms of another, and each must discern what gifts most fully resonate with her sense of self. Adopting this stance allows for the possibility that surrogacy might be fulfilling for one woman and undesirable for another. Yet cultural orientation may also affect a given woman's ability to discern or manifest her charisms. Consider, for instance, a hypothetical culture in which those with power hold the belief that surrogacy is the most highly valued career a woman can choose. If a woman agrees to be a surrogate, then the government of this country will provide her with a home and a stipend so generous that she will become one of the country's most wealthy residents, live in a prestigious neighborhood, and be honored at a national celebration every year. The children she births will be given to women who, in contrast to the surrogate, must raise them without the financial benefits accorded to the surrogate. These women will live in poverty, but, the government explains, they will have the joy of motherhood to satisfy them. A third option will be for the woman to participate in the workforce; if she takes that route, she is by law not allowed to be a mother, and while she will have enough money to meet her basic needs, she will never be prosperous.

In such a culture, a woman is forced to make a choice between valuing her own financial security, valuing a potential maternal instinct, and valuing her identity as a worker. She may decide that while she desperately wants to be a mother or a doctor or a writer, it is more important to take care of her own financial well-being, and so she becomes a surrogate. However, even on the days when the country honors her by name, the woman may wish she had taken a different path. In contrast, another woman may decide to become a mother and wish she had invested more in her professional identity by becoming a worker. In such a culture, the choices offered disable the individual woman, for while the woman is given the appearance of choice, it is essentially ersatz. It appears to be freely made but in fact derives from systemic constraints and constructs, whereas a genuine choice can be made without significant impact from those forces. The woman must therefore make a false choice in this hypothetical culture in light of the priorities of the system in which she operates and must choose between embodying her own charisms and maintaining her own security. As a result, she may be more likely to make a choice, in essence, to exert agency in a way that alienates her from her sense of self and the charisms it comprises.

Examining the effects of the hypothetical culture on the woman drives home the conclusion that humans, surrogates included, do not make choices in a vacuum but rather decide both superficial and important matters with reference to the system in which they participate. With regard to surrogacy, then, it may be reductive to conclude that carrying a growing infant for others to raise must always harm or always provide a good to the surrogate without reference to the overarching cultural dynamics that affect her. Perhaps a more productive line of questioning in an overall evaluation of surrogacy as it affects the surrogate's sense of self is therefore not whether surrogacy exists in a form that does or does not alienate the surrogate's self but what is at stake for the self if surrogacy is practiced under the most ideal circumstances.

Taking a page from surrogates' own description of their experiences, one can understand the surrogate as a social hero, with heroic status being defined by the presence of five characteristics.[21] First, the social hero undertakes a long-term project, as opposed to a military hero who makes a one-time sacrifice bound by a professional code of conduct, such as saving a comrade in the line of fire, or a civilian who makes a short-term sacrifice without being bound to do so, such as saving someone from a burning car. Second, the social hero is either trying to preserve a value that seems to be threatened or is trying to establish a new set of values through the manifestation of heroic imagination.[22] Third, the social hero makes a sacrifice despite the presence of barriers, and fourth, the social hero engages in an act of altruism. Finally, the social hero undertakes the role without obligation.[23]

These characteristics mirror surrogates' self-assessment of their contributions as delineated in the prior chapter: their service takes the better part of a year, or more in cases where the initial insemination fails or where they serve on multiple occasions; they want to allow others to experience the good of parenthood; they undertake the physical difficulty of pregnancy, ultimately willing to give the baby whom they've gestated to others, and, under ideal conditions, they freely agree to do so.

One might respond that the surrogate is not purely altruistic because she receives remuneration for her participation in the pregnancy, and the financial gains outweigh the other-directed nature of the procedure. Second, feminists may be concerned that the altruistic intention of social heroism runs the risk of pressuring women to engage in self-sacrifice in such a way that they necessarily enter into subservient or dependent roles. In response to the first concern, while some surrogates may be more motivated by their own financial gain than they are by altruism, the question here is not whether it is possible or beneficial for a surrogate to be motivated by self-interest but whether the surrogate is vulnerable to self-alienation if she is motivated by altruism. Moreover, the surrogate may be equally self-motivated and altruistically motivated, such that altruism is not canceled out by personal gain. Finally—and perhaps most important to note—altruism and remuneration are not categorically opposed to one another: one might be motivated by altruism to do any number of things and still receive payment.[24] In response to the latter concern, again, at stake is not whether it is possible for the surrogate to experience harm or degradation but why it would be significant if she does not. If some feminists respond that such a query seems too much of a thought experiment, then it is perhaps worthwhile to return to the self-reports of surrogates who, across cultures, report instances where satisfaction characterizes their experiences and where harm does not appear to play a role.[25]

If the surrogate is able to participate in the procedure as a social hero, then it becomes possible to ask whether so doing allows her to remain free from self-alienation, which requires the preclusion of alienation from the three self components—namely, body, desire, and agency. As social hero, the surrogate is willing—or freely expresses desire—to accept the risks of the procedure, risks that can potentially harm the body during the course of the pregnancy, perhaps leaving her with long-term health complications or even her own future infertility (but this is certainly not a given, as a risk does not necessarily correlate with a universal outcome). Second, as social hero, the surrogate acts with no sense of obligation to others, meaning that if she chooses to participate, her choice is motivated by desire rather than external pressures. Likewise, the lack of obligation means that the will to enact her desires remains unaffected by external influence such that agency is maintained. In such a scenario then, where the surrogate functions as social hero, it is possible for her to participate in assisted reproduction in a way that is not self-alienating but that rather affirms the self and its unique charisms.

The surrogate as social hero is, of course, only one construction of surrogacy; however, the goal of this thought experiment was not to narrow what surrogacy can be to one vision but to illustrate one possibility for how self-alienation can be avoided.[26]

Form Two:
Community Alienation and the Surrogate

The condition that arguably plays the most significant role in the negative evaluation of surrogacy is community alienation. Surrogates tend to feel betrayed when relationships with intended parents either go unacknowledged or proceed in ways that counter their expectations, and they experience harm when members of the reproductive community treat them as objects rather than subjects. Surrogates also place great value on actions that parents take to show they are aware of the relationship between them, whether in the form of a gift, an invitation to the family's home, or a heartfelt thank-you note. These acts simultaneously acknowledge the role that surrogates play in the reproductive process while showing that intended parents seek to uphold the surrogate's subjectivity.

Anthropological research across cultures shows that surrogates want their community to acknowledge not only the relationships they share with intended parents but also the specific contributions they make to the reproductive process. They do not want to be named as parents, nor do they seek parental responsibilities, and they do not want the children they birth for intended parents to have the same kind of relationship with them that they share with the children they parent. Rather, they desire validation for their identity as surrogates, or in theological language, they want to be known for the specific charism they bring to reproduction. To eschew communal alienation, then, is to ask the wider community to name and uphold the surrogate for who she desires to be and who she becomes in her reproductive identity.[27]

This kind of acknowledgment becomes possible when the wider community constructs reproduction such a way that the surrogate no longer appears as a threat to parental identity, thereby highlighting the role that a culture's orientation toward reproduction has on the enactment of individual surrogacy experiences. The surrogate, therefore, does not undertake her work or her understanding of it in a vacuum any more than parents make the decision to hire a surrogate in isolation. Cultural values affect both sets of individuals, values that are collectively derived and upheld by a community that extends far beyond either the surrogate or the intended parents. A surrogate's experience of community alienation may therefore hinge upon the reproductive values that the society she lives in constructs: the biblical matriarch Sarah, for instance, existed in a culture that viewed slaves as expendable and without agency such that she could force Hagar's impregnation. American society similarly systemically disregards the bodies, desires, and agency of many of its members—such as minoritized populations, immigrants, those who live in poverty, and persons with physical, cognitive, or psychological disabilities—thereby facilitating experiences of literal and metaphoric surrogacy that say less about their charisms than about the power of systemic abuse.[28]

The orientation of a given culture and its ability to create structures that uphold the three self-components of individual members thereby affects the potential for communal alienation of the surrogate. Cultures that treat the surrogate as object instead of subject prevent the expression of desire, block the exercise of agency, and condone bodily abuse. Cultures that rank individual members by utility as opposed to inherent dignity also permit such maltreatment, maltreatment made even more likely in cases where the surrogate comes from a place of contextual vulnerability wrought by race, economics, sex, or other factors that may be ranked hierarchically within the society.

Form Three: Divine–Human Alienation and the Surrogate

The two departures of Hagar into the wilderness in the Genesis story show God engaging with Hagar in two different ways: in the first, God suggests Hagar return to a seemingly abusive environment, whereas in the second, God provides support for the difficult task of wilderness survival. These may seem contradictory regarding the coherence of divine identity, as God in the first passage appears to condone abuse, and God in the second advocates for at least a degree of liberation.[29] God's reaction to Hagar's surrogacy thereby complicates an interpretation of the surrogate experience itself, and the reader is left asking whether surrogacy for Hagar was, in the end, in the service of perpetuating abuse (the first departure) or in the service of facilitating freedom to any degree (the second departure).

One way to parse the discrepancy would be to consider the significance of time in regard to its relationship to process: time binds the human experience, its limits shaping mortality and its progress allowing for growth. Processes therefore are inevitably time bound, as are stories, which have a beginning, middle, and end. Human development hinges upon this relationship: time allows the individual to engage in the process of growth, be it in the physical growth of childhood in the development of the brain or in the cultivation of wisdom, so that time along with process allows for growth.

Hagar's life existed within the bounds of time, and her experience of surrogacy was limited by the constraints of seconds, minutes, hours, days, and years. As a result, surrogacy for Hagar has multiple meanings, depending on which time one references. At its earliest, Hagar's rape presents as an evil, as does Sarah's subsequent abusiveness. Her second departure, however, adds a new layer to surrogacy because possibilities for freedom and liberation begin to emerge: only in the wilderness does Hagar speak; only in the wilderness can Hagar exert agency, absent the tyrannical influence of Sarah and Abraham. As a result, surrogacy becomes an ambivalent opportunity for a better life than Hagar may have had otherwise—unless, of course, one stops to question why God allows such suffering in the first place.

However, rather than running down the rabbit hole of theodicy, one can ask, "What now?"[30] Given that Hagar was raped, given that Hagar became a surrogate, what is needed in response within the confines of the divine-human relationship is the question of concern, not only systematically but also pastorally. An acknowledgment of the intersection of time and process may help in this regard, because the passing of time is necessary in human experience, from what we know from psychological investigations of human nature to the construction of meaning in the aftermath of trauma. Meaning does not appear immediately, nor is meaning constructed as a static entity, but evolves and grows in depth with time. Acknowledging the intersection of time and process as one way that God engages in relationship with humans in the aftermath of suffering is therefore also to recognize that possibility cannot open without process and that process does not—at least within the boundaries of our current mortal form—occur without time. Insofar as divine–human alienation is concerned, then, Hagar's departures seem to indicate that engaging with God over time is essential for anyone who suffers—in this case, the surrogate—to counter alienation.

Divine alienation, therefore, may be posited to occur when process appears static and when time, while passing, appears stationary in terms of growth and change. Such a state disrupts a fundamental element of God's creation—that we are meant to exist not within stagnancy but within time that facilitates process. This hypothesis may help to loosen some of the ambivalence around Hagar's two departures as well as the ambivalence around the reasons that contemporary surrogates volunteer to offer their wombs for the creation of new life: as time-bound creatures, both Hagar and the contemporary surrogate find themselves enmeshed in concrete problems that must be responded to in order to prevent a perpetual static state of being.[31] The concrete problem may be survival, liberation, restoration, or salvation, but a given problem cannot be said to be resolved—nor a given evil defeated—without an appropriate response to the process as it relates to a given point in time. Divine engagement is therefore engagement that responds to the problem at hand, be it a problem that requires the need for survival, liberation, or something else entirely. In turn, divine–human alienation occurs when systemic or individual forces attempt to maintain stasis. Such stasis violates the created order precisely because time continues to advance while process, its rightful companion, is restrained, and as a result, opportunities for problem solving experience restraint as well.

Consider, by way of example, the case of Genie. Genie—whose name is a pseudonym—was born in 1957 and was a victim of severe physical abuse. Her father, who believed that she was intellectually disabled, locked Genie away from other members of the household and immobilized her by strapping her to a toilet or to a crib. Genie experienced severe social deprivation during this time, to the point that she did not develop basic language skills. The state of California intervened in her case when Genie was thirteen years old, and in the aftermath of her discovery, Genie became a research subject for psychologists and linguists, who were interested in figuring out how the brain responded to such severe linguistic deprivation.[32]

Genie's case highlights the integration of time and process and the way in which alienation can be defined by the deprivation of process for the purpose of maintaining stasis.[33] Genie was unable to engage in basic processes of human development because of the way that her father attempted to keep her, literally, in a state of stasis. It could be argued that while evil occurred in the form of abuse, evil also occurred because the act of abuse attempted to prevent time and process from coexisting, thereby affecting Genie's ability to act as a self. The evil in such a case, then, is not confined to the event itself but to its aftermath and to the effects of the event on the self and the self's ability to develop into the fullness of God's hopes for it.

If one extrapolates this hypothesis to Hagar's experience of surrogacy, one might say that divine–human alienation occurred prior to both of Hagar's departures and during the time when she was confined in a static state of being as a slave in Sarah and Abraham's tribe. However, at both points in the wilderness, divine–human alienation ceases, as God engages with Hagar to solve the immediate problem, thereby allowing time and process to once again move together.

Form One:
Self-Alienation and Surrogate Children

Children have thus far received minimal attention in this work, and yet their creation is the purported purpose of surrogacy, and their worldview may well be affected by their origins. Unlike the adults who participate in the procedures, however, the children birthed through them cannot share their opinions during the process of deciding whether to engage a third party in reproduction or during the earliest stages of their development. It is the participating adults who make decisions on behalf of this developing human, prior to conception and in utero. Indeed, some may never know about the involvement of a surrogate in their creation.

The question of what self-alienation could look like for children thus depends on what kind of opportunities they are given to develop various components of the self. Consider the body in a scenario where a child is not told about the use of a traditional surrogate in reproduction, meaning a surrogate who provides her own egg in addition to her womb for procreation. If the child is raised to believe that his body emerged from the genetics of his mother and father, then he may have various false conceptions about it—he may believe that he has a propensity for illnesses on his mother's side or that he is right-handed because his mother is right-handed or that he will be short like his mother. In a more serious variant, the child may believe that his mother will have a high probability of being a bone marrow match after he learns that he has leukemia. Each example illustrates the way that the child's lack of access to information about his body affects his perception of it in ways that alienate him from the truth about its origins and functions.[34]

Similar arguments may be made concerning the other two self components, desire and agency. Desire for social belonging—or a desire for relationships—serves as one of several root desires for the individual, along with physiological, safety, esteem, and self-actualization needs. The self therefore seeks to be in relationship with others as a means of facilitating social belonging, with the family often having the most formative influence on the self's development. These influences, however, best serve the individual self when they seek to uphold other self components: the parents who abuse and lock a child in a room communicate negative messages about the child's social belonging in the family that in turn affect her esteem, sense of safety, and ability to achieve self-actualization, and likely also her understanding of embodiment and agency. This example illustrates how social belonging must occur in a way that validates the self as a social being in order to promote the self's overall health and must be undertaken with an authentic desire to accept that self into the social unit without seeking to deconstruct the authentic expression of any of its components.

Self-alienation may occur in surrogacy when children are not offered authentic opportunities to engage in social belonging, including the opportunity to construct a relationship with the surrogate. Conversations with parents, the surrogate, and children about what it means to have been carried in utero by a surrogate or to share the surrogate's genetic material become particularly important as a result; giving children a chance to participate in these conversations offers them a chance to discern and express what healthy social belonging looks like and to express their root desire for it while also exercising agency to enact it. The support that surrogates and parents can offer the child in the task of seeking social belonging, then, becomes an opportunity for the child to more fully understand what it means to be a self with both root desire and agency.[35]

This process cannot occur, however, when children are not told about or do not have access to their origins.[36] The potential for self-alienation in children birthed by a surrogate is therefore contingent upon the attitudes and decisions of the adults who participated in the procedure prior to the child's cognizance. In such cases, the root story of their creation is a lie manufactured by these adults, thereby constructing the self of the child as a lie as well.

Self-alienation therefore occurs in situations where children do not know of or cannot meet the participants who contributed to their creation. This understanding of self-alienation not only supports the development of various self components but also is reinforced by data about the psychological wellness of children who are adopted or who had a gamete donor. Studies illustrate that adopted children struggle with their sense of identity when they are not told of their birth parents' existence, leading the domestic adoption industry to by and large embrace open adoptions where intended parents meet the birth ones and either children have an ongoing relationship with the latter set of adults under preset parameters or the birth parents' identity is kept in records that children may access at a certain age. Recent studies done with children of anonymous egg and sperm donors are now yielding similar findings. Individuals who are not raised with knowledge of or access to the identities of their donor gametes may experience psychological struggles related to self-concept because of assumptions about who they are in relation to their parents. One might infer that similar questions about identity could emerge for surrogate children.[37]

Two anthropological conclusions thus emerge. First, the self gets constituted in community so that deprivation of community becomes a source of self-alienation and community engagement becomes a source of restoration. Second, the self has a right to know its origins such that deprivation of that knowledge constitutes a source of self-alienation. Practices that create reproductive communities where children both know about the existence of and can cultivate relationships with surrogates or donors can productively address both of these dangers.

Form Two: Community Alienation and Surrogate Children

As chapter 1 explained, an individual's reproductive story begins in childhood, with young children practicing different manifestations of the self that may one day become realities. Children develop these hypothetical imaginings with reference to their own experience and to the stories they hear about reproduction and parenthood, and the selves they test out are often shaped through their own experiences. It therefore becomes crucial for parents and the wider community to actively involve children in this process as agents who are capable of exerting subjectivity and naming desires.

One might object that children may find knowledge of or a relationship with the surrogate confusing or suggest that it will jeopardize the identity of the mother. Moreover, parents may not want their children to think of themselves as different from other children or think that their mother is not a real mother because she did not carry them. As a result, adults in the reproductive process may try to craft the child's birth narrative in such a way as to ameliorate these concerns.

While such actions are undertaken in the interest of children, they fail to include the children in the narrative process, instead relying on the needs and experiences of adults to structure how the children will ultimately understand their own identities and the shape of their reproductive selves. This denies the agency of the child while simultaneously projecting the desires of other members of the reproductive community onto them. Such practices therefore serve as examples of how community alienation can occur when the community affects the child's understanding of surrogacy in a way that negatively affects the child's self, specifically in regard to agency.

One might follow up by asking what kind of relationship a child and surrogate ought to have: perhaps the child should think of the surrogate as a second mother, or perhaps the surrogate should treat the child as a friend. But perhaps the attempt to circumscribe relationships is what leads to relational difficulties, because attempting to delineate the specifics of how people should relate to one another presumes a degree of similarity between individuals that may not exist. By the same token, failing to circumscribe relationships creates a permissive environment that allows for nefarious activity. Perhaps, then, the way to avoid community alienation is not to micromanage relationships nor to permit all behaviors between individuals but to encourage members of the reproductive community to construct relationships that uphold and strengthen the body, desire, and agency of members in collaboration with one another. In so doing, these members help each other to construct the self in its fullness, including helping to construct the reproductive story.

This process may be tempting to avoid in regard to children: adults may believe children lack the knowledge and experience to have valid opinions about what family relationships ought to look like. Yet discarding the opinions or inclinations of children outright may undermine the child's agency, in essence suggesting that the child is somehow less than a full self by virtue of age.[38] The cycle of evaluating an individual based on certain skills or assets rather than the presence of self components thereby perpetuates itself, teaching children from a young age that utility matters more than intrinsic value and that they must reach certain milestones or at least a certain birthday in order to be, in essence, fully human. In order to avoid community alienation, then, it becomes important to integrate children into conversations about the kind of relationships they want to have with members of their reproductive community, and it becomes the responsibility of adults in the community to acknowledge the children's wishes, while assisting them in making choices either with them or on their behalf that facilitate the development of self components.

Form Three: Divine–Human Alienation and Surrogate Children

The children birthed through surrogates may function as a theodicy solution for the parents who inaugurated the process, and as such their birth projects a purpose onto them: they exist as the fulfillment of the parental reproductive narrative. One might propose, then, that divine–human alienation is an impossibility for children if viewed from the perspective of parents; however, the projected meaning itself may be a source of divine–human alienation if a child's own narrative is dictated by that of the parents, for it would deprive the child of a chance to construct the self apart from the parents' projection onto it. That self may be constructed in relationship with others, but this is different from having the self components imposed by outside sources, which would deprive the child of the chance to exert agency in the service of self development.

It is possible to relate this back to the possibility that divine–human alienation occurs for the surrogate when time and process are not allowed to coexist such that stasis dominates movement. The child, like the surrogate, may also exist in stasis if the child is not permitted to embody an authentic self, perhaps because others have attempted to project a self onto the child or perhaps because the child has not received information about his or her origins that would allow for the possibility of authentic self embodiment.

If divine–human alienation occurs when time and process are not allowed to coexist, then one might surmise that alienation occurs for surrogate children who experience imposed stasis that prevents them from moving toward an authentic embodiment of the self, as might be the case if external forces prevent authentic self embodiment either through projection or obstruction. Ishmael's experiences in the wilderness may offer additional insights into what divine–human alienation for the child looks like: the pregnant Hagar hears the message of an angel of the Lord in the first departure in Gen 16, an angel who makes promises that relate to Ishmael's life but ones that Ishmael does not yet inhabit. It is only in Genesis 21:20 that the text presents God in direct relationship with Ishmael, stating that God remained with Ishmael in the wilderness as he gained the skills he needed to survive and to thrive, as Ishmael eventually married and birthed twelve sons who became tribal chiefs. Ishmael therefore did not experience direct solidarity with God within the confines of Abraham's tribe but instead participated in that solidarity only when he was able to escape from the confines of the tribe's identity and establish his own community.

For the child of surrogacy, then, the potential for divine–human alienation emerges when the child feels unable to move toward this authentic self embodiment, or in theological terms, when the child's identity becomes enmeshed with the parental vision for the self without the possibility of the child's own input as to whether that self is desired. Such a vision, at its broadest, represents the basis of any coming-of-age story—children develop a sense of self by being able to imagine and experiment with potential selves, in turn discerning the utility and purpose of the body, desires for the present or future, and how to act to achieve them. When this process cannot be undertaken, then the child may be said to exist in a state of stasis that alienates the self from that which God intends the child to discover and inhabit.

Conclusion

The corporate affects the individual in self-enhancing or self-defeating ways, challenging what is at stake theologically for that individual. Yet individuals exist in networks of relationships, one network being that of families, such that to limit analysis of surrogacy to the individual would be to neglect theological consideration of what is at stake for the unit that surrogacy ultimately seeks to create. What the family is and how membership within it is determined is therefore affected by any given theology of the self, in turn affecting who is an insider, who exists on the borders, and who is beyond the boundaries of familial inclusion.

5

Consonant Dependency Care as a New Vision for Family

Humans cannot survive without connection. It is unlikely that a given person, alone, can procure enough food to thrive while simultaneously maintaining a shelter, stitching clothes, and caring for his or her young. Relationships therefore emerge from both a need for connection with others and the ability of others to help a single person obtain what cannot be achieved in isolation. Units ranging from the nuclear family to tribes to nations capitalize on this connective basis: a son needs his mother to meet his basic needs; some members of a tribe defend assets while others hunt; factory workers sew a blouse that an executive purchases at a premium so that she does not have to sew her own.

Connection between humans is not only evident from practice but also reflected in biblical formulations about interhuman and divine-human relationships. Genesis 1:28 emphasizes that God shares an image connection with humans; Isaiah 49:15 states that God cannot forsake humans any more than a mother can abandon her own child; Psalm 71:6 says that humans rely on God from birth; and Jeremiah 1:5 states that God knows humans from before conception. Matthew 28:20 closes with Jesus' promise to be with the disciples until the end of days, and Paul describes humans in Romans 8:16 as God's children and in Ephesians 1:5 as specifically adopted children of God. A plain reading of the biblical text could thereby be said to propose, through a variety of logical permutations, that God's self exists in continual, sustaining relationship within the persons of the Trinity, so that Christianity potentially insists that to be human is to be connected to God and to other humans who are made in God's image.

That this connection is foundational to Christianity is therefore not a new claim, nor is it a new claim to apply to the family, which some Christian traditions describe as the interhuman set of relationships with the greatest potential to mirror the divine–human one.[1] But even if one sets Christian traditions aside, the family is the unit of individuals to whom Americans tend to believe they owe the most in terms of love, loyalty, and resources. Perhaps that is why the family often becomes the locus of discussions about the significance and health of relationships in society at large: if this primary set of relationships falters, then it could follow that the stability of other relationships may falter as well. Family matters thus become contentious societal matters, because if the family is the fundamental shaper of societal norms, then to change the structure of the family is to challenge the norms on which society builds and maintains itself. Arguments become increasingly heated when faith factors in: when one believes that family is preordained by God, is the most intimate way that humans practice their faith, and is necessary for the proper exercise of Christianity and the overall health of society, then families become a battleground for those who seek to shape a given culture.

Political debates over the past fifty years provide evidence to this effect. The invention of the birth control pill, a greater acceptance of sex before and outside of marriage, the wider use of and greater societal tolerance of divorce, and women's increasing role in the workplace all fueled debates about family values that came to a head in the 1970s and 1980s. Christian conservatives and their representative politicians railed against policies and cultural norms that threatened the survival of the two-parent, married, heterosexual household, concerns that took on a new dimension as the conversation shifted to the legality and morality of same-sex marriage in the new millennium. Such conversations about the formulation of families remain culturally charged precisely because Americans attribute great import to the family as the locus of development of moral values, discovery of divine blessing and revelation, and personal self-fulfillment. It is worthwhile, then, to consider how surrogacy affects the family, not just in regard to its individual members but in regard to family as a unit.

Social Belonging as the Basis of Family

Family provides a primary way that humans engage in connections, with some of their most intimate being fostered between parents and children. So when couples cannot create children through heterosexual intercourse, they find themselves unable to manifest the kinds of relationships that they believe give positive meaning to life. The drive to use third-party reproduction, however, exists not just because of a desire to create new relationships but also because of an unspoken societal desire to perpetuate the genes of the parents. The patriarchal understanding of reproduction as a genetic connection maintains prominence over the relational understanding of reproduction that historically originated with the contributions of pregnant women. Assisted reproduction provides the possibility that individuals who cannot achieve the biological family norm through intercourse alone might achieve the closest possible alternative, be it a biological family brought about through in vitro fertilization involving the gametes of both parents or a third-party procedure that uses only the gametes of one. The use of a surrogate further drives home the commitment to biological family as the family norm because a surrogate, whose body protects the genes of one or both members of the couple, helps the intended parents more closely equate themselves to the norm than they could otherwise. The relationship provided by the surrogate's womb, meanwhile, is subordinate to a parental genetic link.

What third-party procedures such as surrogacy highlight is a societal desire to use the heterosexual biological family as the reference class to which other family structures seek to equate themselves. Equality, then, gets defined by sameness, by the ability of parties to achieve identical ends, and so when sameness is impossible, the closest possible alternative becomes the next best thing.[2] Assisted reproduction therefore provides an opportunity for couples to attain that which associates as closely as possible to the biological family norm. Indeed, the very existence of such reproductive technologies as surrogacy points to the desire on the part of individuals to maintain their genetic lineage and therefore their relationship to the biological family norm; otherwise there would be no market for in vitro fertilization, gamete donation, or surrogacy in the first place, given that adoption has been a long-standing alternative.[3]

Several problems exist with this construction. In particular, attempts to use third-party reproduction in order to achieve the biological family norm constrain the narrative capability of those who experience infertility and reproductive loss. As chapter 1 summarized, psychological literature about trauma generally, and reproductive trauma specifically, illustrates that healing occurs when individuals are given an opportunity to regain control through the creation of a narrative that integrates the trauma into the overarching meaning of life, even as the supremacy of the biological family facilitates the implicit conclusion that the "correct" end to a story of infertility or reproductive loss involves the creation of something that mimics it. This constrains the narrative process. Instead of allowing individuals to discern what ending feels most appropriate to them, they find themselves at best influenced and at worst pressured to achieve a given one—namely, to manifest a family that perpetuates their genetic lineage.[4] In other words, if the reproductive narrative were a Choose Your Own Adventure book, cultural assumptions—and not individual adults—would dictate which adventure to take.[5]

Such pressure has implications for self-concept. If desire is indeed a key grounding point of the self, then constraints on root desire constitute an attempt to pressure, harm, or even annihilate it. However, if reproductive capabilities are not essential to human identity, then one might well ask whether reproduction can function as a root desire. Here, perhaps, it makes most sense to understand the root desire for children not as a desire for reproduction but rather as part of a broader root desire for social belonging. In this case, social belonging means a set of embodied relationships through which an individual can participate in the ongoing construction of the self in community, alongside others who are committed to that individual's self construction, just as that individual simultaneously commits to theirs.[6] Especially in a culture such as that of white, upper-middle-class America—which is not the only culture within the United States but is the one that uses assisted reproduction the most—the primacy of the nuclear family, the erosion of social institutions, including the church, and the rise of social media as a method to develop disembodied relationships have created a greater need for a such social belonging. It is not children, then, that are necessarily required for the human to satisfy this need. Rather, the experience of wanting for children, biological or otherwise, may be said to function as a projected desire that emerges from the root desire for social belonging in general. When there is pressure to believe that biological children are somehow superior to other forms of relationship, then it becomes difficult for individuals to exercise the root desire for social belonging in the way that is most authentic to them, precisely because biological children may function as an idol or a pinnacle to be achieved rather than a desire to be fulfilled. In other words, it may well be the case that the projected desire for children is healthy and life-giving; however, when root desire cannot freely realize because society's conception of proper relationships and the role of family function as a kind of colored lens through which individuals see in order to construct their relationships, and in turn their selves, then projected desire may just as easily become less salutary. The same would be true if society overemphasized the importance of adoption or childless living, because each would prevent the individual from engaging in a process of free and unconstrained self-reflection about root desire.[7]

The economic structures of a given society may further agitate or reinforce the individual's ability to freely discern how to transmit root desire into agency. In the United States, for instance, it is rarely if ever more cost effective to hire a surrogate than to reproduce by other means; however, other forms of assisted reproduction—specifically artificial insemination and in vitro fertilization—may be covered by insurance, thereby influencing the decision to adopt. A couple may save thousands of dollars by trying to reproduce biologically, even taking into account the federal tax credit for adoption, and so while they may desire children by any means—not necessarily biological ones—economic policies that favor biological reproduction may sway them to pursue one option over another and affect how they materialize root desire as agency.

Structural constraints related to time may also come into play. Couples who want to reproduce via a surrogate in the United States can—under ideal circumstances—complete the process within a year, whereas those who choose to adopt face not only an uncertain time line but also additional evaluative measures, like home studies, that other forms of family creation do not require. Indeed, adoption is the only form of long-term family creation that requires external approval of individuals' economic means and moral character.[8] One might argue, and perhaps appropriately, that birth parents have a right to know the conditions into which they commit their biological offspring, thus justifying the extended requirements. The result, however, is a hurdle for intended parents that can be avoided with the use of reproductive technology so that the desire to adopt becomes impinged by the reality that assisted reproduction involves less gatekeeping, which becomes especially significant to older intended parents who are also more likely to experience reproductive difficulties.

A twofold set of concerns therefore emerges when one assumes that the biological family is an autonomous one to which others should seek to equate themselves: First, it is a falsehood. No family is autonomous, because an egg needs sperm and a hospitable environment in which to unite and grow—thereby delineating the use of at least two participants in the reproductive process, and during pregnancy, the couple also need medicines and vitamins crafted by scientists, as well as doctors, midwives, nurses and extended family who provide medical and social support. The creation of another human being, therefore, always requires connection. All reproduction could rightly be termed "assisted."

Second, the autonomous, biological family ideal renders inferior those adults that depend on others more explicitly to create family structures or those who choose to remain childless themselves, and it judges inferior the children who emerge from alternative arrangements. If the adults involved cannot form a family in the privileged way, then that can reflect negatively on the entire family unit, and as argued in chapter 1, it is anthropologically problematic to assess the value of the self via reproductive capabilities of the body because the body, while a key component of the self, is rightly evaluated on the inherent dignity of the whole and not by the function of its parts. To advocate for the autonomous biological family as the superlative family model is therefore to implicitly judge inferior the selves of those who cannot reproduce. This creates a hierarchy of adults, ranking those whose bodies have certain capabilities and those whose bodies do not, a hierarchy that can be exploited so that those who do not ascend it become vulnerable to those who do, realized through various forms of exploitation or domination.[9] Practices of secrecy serve as a case study here: adults may not tell children they were adopted or birthed through gamete donation or surrogacy in order to preserve their own status as biologically based parents. However, children who are not told of their origins can struggle with questions of identity later in life because they do not have access to the fullness of who they are or feel a sense of betrayal that stable relationships with their parents are built on false foundations. The illusion of the autonomous family can therefore lead to practices that cause contagious harm in the name of preserving an institution of supposed good.[10]

Such possibilities for exploitation flow in multiple directions in surrogacy arrangements: news stories about surrogates in developing countries such as India illustrate the kinds of harms that surrogates can experience at the hands of intended parents and medical professionals. However, intended parents themselves may face exploitation when they enter a doctor's office with photos of live babies on the walls—thereby exploiting their unrealized hopes through their pocketbooks—or when medical professionals again and again offer the hope of biological children in order to achieve personal gain while neglecting to mention the possibility of adoption or childless living with the same enthusiasm.[11] Intended parents can also face potential exploitation from surrogates because of the theoretical—and hopefully not realized—threat that they could harm or withhold the baby. Hence, the possibility for exploitation can stem from judging inferior the bodies of those who cannot reproduce or favoring the biological family model.

One could counter that defining family by relationship alone jeopardizes the human race, with the Shakers emblematizing just such an outcome. The Shakers decreased in number to the point of eradicating themselves when they as a collective chose to eschew sexual relations and rely on adoption alone to perpetuate the religion. Biology, therefore, must play its part. Yet to say that biology is essential to family's identity is like saying that an ingredient in a recipe defines the final product. Pizza can function as an example: a pizza is never the same as a sugar cookie. One is usually savory, with a crust base and some permutation of toppings; the other is sweet and usually served as dessert. That said, pizza does not require a specific ingredient in order to maintain its overall integrity. The crust may be made of white flour, whole wheat flour, or even rice flour or cauliflower; the toppings may or may not include sauce and cheese; and other possible toppings such as spinach, pepperoni, or mushrooms may enhance the pie's flavor profile. Pizza, therefore, is defined less by a specific ingredient or set of ingredients than it is by its form as a crust with toppings. Side by side, these different pizza manifestations are still clearly identifiable as pizza, and though a single bite into each demonstrates their varied flavors, they all fit within its Platonic ideal. In that way, pizza maintains its integrity as an identifiable form that is separate from foods like bread (a base with no toppings) or tomato sauce (topping with no base). By analogy, the passing of genes—through intercourse or through human manipulation—is necessary for the creation of another human being just as the crust is a necessary component of pizza. But forming another human being by linking genes together is not the same as forming a family. The family binds a human being into a social belonging unit, so that the family can take different biological forms while still maintaining its integrity, just as pizza may be composed of different permutations of ingredients but still be considered pizza.

An argument that overstresses the role of biology therefore assumes that increasing the validity afforded one definition of family—the biological family—necessitates decreasing the status of another. In other words, just because the human species needs biological reproduction does not mean that it does not need relationships, and indeed, a biological connection to another human being without love is nothing more than the scientific fact of shared genes. Relationships must play their part. Hence, to define family by relationship is not to say that biology becomes irrelevant but rather to say that biology alone does not a family make. This definition gives relationships primacy, arguing that they are the foremost facilitators of social belonging, supported by various permutations of genetics.[12]

Defining the family as a unit of social belonging as opposed to a unit based in genetic similarity recognizes the significance of relationships to human identity because, while genetics inform the mechanics of the body, it is relationships that construct the fullness of the self. This definition therefore uplifts the significance of relationships and downplays autonomy in relation to both self construction and family definition. The family, therefore, is not made up of autonomous humans who share a genetic connection but rather by selves who mutually construct one another's identity. Defining the family as primarily a unit of social belonging also allows for more expansive configurations than the biological family model allows, thereby removing the biological family as the reference class that other forms of family ought to imitate.[13] It also prevents the temptation of seeing those who cannot reproduce as somehow instrumentally impaired, instead opening the possibility for recognizing their intrinsic wholeness while also opening the possibility for multiple family constructions that can have equal value.[14]

The Danger of Equality as Sameness in Surrogacy

Thinking of family as a unit defined by the shared quest for social belonging and the activity of mutual identity construction has implications for intended parents, surrogates, and children. If these constituents are understood to be autonomous individuals by virtue of their freedom or power to act—and, in turn, their freedom to autonomously constitute the self—then surrogacy becomes permissible under conditions where participants can freely choose to participate. Such is an argument from the perspective of liberal philosophy or ethics.[15] However, if one starts with the dual premises of a socially constructed self and a family unit dedicated to that process of construction—views that might be best situated within the framework of care ethics—then the boundaries of permissible surrogacy and the understanding of the relationships between those individuals look different.[16] The starting point becomes the recognition that the self is fundamentally dependent on other selves for its needs to be met, be they practical needs or identity-construction needs. This in turn requires acknowledging a certain degree of individual vulnerability, because the individual is no longer presumed to be able to autonomously meet various needs but rather is dependent on others for those needs to be met.

An awareness of vulnerability takes on even more significance with reference to those who want to start families but who experience infertility or reproductive loss: these individuals must depend on others to help them construct their identity as parents. However, if the biological family is the norm or reference class they seek to join, then the vulnerability wrought by infertility or reproductive loss takes on a further dimension insofar as they are unable to fully attain membership in the reference class, although assisted reproduction, in all its various forms, helps them get closer than they might otherwise. In other words, those who experience infertility or reproductive loss and who use surrogates to bear children appear, to some extent, to be holding their experiences of family creation to the biological family norm, since the surrogate allows them to achieve the greatest possible degree of sameness with biological families. If the intended mother's womb is unequipped to carry the biological offspring of both intended parents, then at least the surrogate can do that. If both intended parents do not have reproductive gametes that are up to the task of joining together, then at least one intended parent can give his or her own and a donor can be recruited to provide the second. If neither intended parent has usable gametes, then at least donors who physically resemble both can be chosen. Surrogacy therefore affords those who experience infertility and reproductive loss the opportunity to approach the norm of the genetic family that defines the reference class. However, it does not allow these individuals to achieve the ideal because the only way to do that would be for the couple to be able to bear biological children conceived through sex and carried by a member of the couple, a task their bodies are unable to achieve. In other words, in vitro fertilization, gamete donation, and surrogacy all help the infertile couple to move toward sameness with the biological family model that serves as the reference class; however, that approximation of sameness does not correlate with equality.[17]

Surrogacy partially fails in its attempt to achieve equality through sameness because full sameness would require some solution to infertility and reproductive loss that allows for complete manifestation of the biological family model, and this, at least with current technology, cannot be achieved. A family created through surrogacy will never be the same as a family that originated a different way. All parties—intended parents, surrogate, and children—are affected by the unique contours of surrogacy in ways that other configurations of family are not. Sameness, therefore, is impossible. However, if sameness is no longer the goal, then its attainment becomes irrelevant.

Applying the Dependency Model to Surrogacy

Infertility and reproductive loss provide evidence of just one type of human experience wherein individuals cannot autonomously manifest desire through agency, rendering them dependent on others to create the family they desire through adoption or third-party reproduction. Here Eva Kittay's notion of dependency work may prove valuable. As Kittay explains it, dependency work occurs when one party—a charge—requires a degree of care while another party—known as the dependency worker—offers the care, but to the detriment of his or her own care. Kittay primarily explains dependency care with reference to children, the elderly, or individuals with profound cognitive or physical disabilities who cannot independently meet the basic needs of daily living. Such individuals necessarily function as charges and require the assistance of dependency workers, who in turn experience vulnerability because by providing care to another, they sacrifice their own ability to provide for themselves and adopt subordinate positions to others who are not responsible for the care of another.[18] The mother who does not take paid work in order to care for her children must rely on her spouse for financial support; the daughter who quits her job to care for her parents needs the state's welfare system; the individual who works as a caretaker for an adult with serious disabilities is subservient to her employer, and given that such work tends to be low paying and minimally respected and typically falls to individuals who have minimal education, the vulnerability of such a worker may be compounded by her social and economic circumstances.

Kittay proposes that the dependency worker's responsibilities to others invalidate conversations about equality that assume that equality occurs with the achievement of sameness precisely because such responsibilities prevent sameness from being possible. The dependency worker will never be the same as the nondependency worker, and so providing the same material circumstances will not in turn make the two parties equal. Moreover, justice for the dependency worker and the nondependency worker cannot be evaluated through the criterion of sameness because these two groups do not face the same realities. The dependency worker's burdens require additional support: a man who is the full-time caretaker for his elderly parents cannot also take paid work and remove himself from the financial constraints imposed by dependency work, just as a woman who stays at home with young children may be unable to return to school and obtain her degree because she does not have money for childcare. Those who serve in dependency positions require an additional level of support, support that they must derive externally because of the constraints they face. This means that the dependency worker is unable to achieve self-support because, while he or she is responsible for the charge, the charge is unable to assist the dependency worker.[19] Kittay therefore suggests that justice for dependency workers requires assistance from those who exist outside the dyad of the dependency worker and the charge: those outside the dependency system must become involved in order for dependency workers to have their own needs met along with those of the charge.[20]

The particular burdens of the dependency worker change the nature of what equality can look like because the existence of the charge negates the possibility that the dependency worker could ever be the same as someone who does not engage in this role. Someone who has the extra burden of care is simply not the same as someone who does not. Kittay therefore shifts the nature of equality away from sameness to redefine it as equal membership in the community.[21] A dependency work formulation cannot be said to be equal where equality is defined as sameness, because the dependency worker still carries the extra burdens imposed by the charge, but it can be said to be equal in a different way: the dependency worker receives in kind what he or she offers. The worker is able to meet the needs of another and in turn finds his or her own needs met by those who can do likewise. For example, consider a woman who has quit her job to engage in full-time care of her sick mother. The woman forgoes her own income in order to meet her mother's basic needs. In Kittay's vision of equality, the dependency worker would receive from the larger community—which is not directly engaged in the care—what she offers to her mother so that the community might provide for her financial needs as well as for any other personal responsibilities she cannot engage in because she cares for her mother.[22] The dependency worker in this community would not be the same as a woman who worked and earned her own income; however, the two women could still be considered equal insofar as the community met the needs of each individual.

The Surrogate as Disrupter of Sameness and Blender of Dependency Care

Kittay's work focuses on scenarios in which there is a clearly defined dependency worker and charge and, in turn, a clearly directed focus of care from the worker to a charge who lacks certain abilities and is involuntarily in that position.[23] Kittay does acknowledge scenarios in which dependency workers may function in what she calls an extended sense—though this is not the focus of her analysis—suggesting that individuals such as line cooks, waiters, and administrative assistants fall into this category because they provide dependency care to those who technically could manage without the help but who choose not to.[24] Examples include a person who pays restaurant staff to prepare a meal he could cook himself or a CEO who could clean her own clothes but who sends them to a dry cleaner; in these scenarios of extended dependency care, dependency workers have the capability to do the task at hand but choose to spend time differently and therefore use others to provide for some of their own needs. This extended dependency care differs in significant ways from the narrower definition that Kittay discusses both because it usually takes place in the workplace and because it occurs in public with individuals who could theoretically meet the needs they project onto the dependency worker.[25]

What emerges when seeking to apply the dependency model to surrogacy is the fact that surrogacy fits into neither the narrower nor the extended definitions of care. The surrogate theoretically functions in the workplace because she receives payment for her services, but her work is in many ways undertaken in private. She may never meet the parents with whom she contracts or may lie to family and friends about why she is pregnant, and details about her pregnancy may only be known to herself and her doctors. She also develops the future child within her body, and while she may share elements of the pregnancy experience with others via ultrasounds or by allowing others to touch her belly, there remains an intimacy to pregnancy that belongs to her alone. The work that she undertakes as a surrogate is therefore not only highly personalized but also defined by the relational contribution that historically belonged to women in reproduction: if she is a traditional surrogate, meaning that the egg belongs to her and not a donor, then it becomes difficult to differentiate her role from that of a woman who intends to raise her biological offspring until the point of birth. Both women consent to be the primary relationship source for the fetus while it develops in utero and in turn consent to the role as dependency worker for the duration of the pregnancy. However, the possibility for sameness concludes at birth when the surrogate ceases to function as a dependency worker and the biological mother continues to do so.

And yet, a worker dimension to surrogacy sets it apart from historical conceptions of motherhood even during the pregnancy. A surrogate receives remuneration in the United States—unlike a biological mother—because culture constructs her role in reproduction not as a maternal gift but as work.[26] This would seem to situate her not as any kind of mother but rather as an extended dependency worker who contracts with others to fulfill their desires by obtaining what they choose not to obtain on their own. Such an interpretation makes sense if parenthood is conceived as a choice and not as an essential component of adult identity. If, as chapter 1 argued, reproductive capability is not essential to the self, then the surrogate is not fulfilling a basic need but rather a want.[27] A person can survive, after all, if he or she does not become a parent, but that same person cannot survive independently if both hands are chopped off and no prosthetics exist. Such a person is unable to meet basic needs for survival without the assistance of a dependency worker in the latter scenario, while in the former, the limits imposed by the inability to reproduce are not themselves life-threatening. Even if reproduction is framed by the broader need for social belonging, then one can argue that this need may be met by relationships other than parent–child ones; however, the need may also be met by the surrogate serving as an extended dependency worker.

The conditions of infertility or reproductive loss that drive individuals to hire surrogates may therefore be said to situate the surrogate as an extended dependency worker instead of a mother, yet this too can be challenged by asking whether she is more appropriately conceived of as a charge because of the dynamics and cultural construction of the reproductive process.[28] This argument can be most compellingly made if one construes pregnancy as a disability, yet one need not go so far to make the point.[29] Pregnancy often hampers a woman's physical abilities: she may be unable to physically exert herself at the rate she did prior to pregnancy, find that back pain prevents certain activities, or be unable to touch her own toes. More seriously, pregnancy's nausea and fatigue can be so debilitating that some women need to be hospitalized, and complications from conditions such as preeclampsia, gestational diabetes, and placenta accreta that develop in later trimesters can endanger the life of the woman herself or raise the risk of health issues following the baby's birth. It is the pregnant woman, then, who finds herself in a place of vulnerability and perhaps in need of dependency care.

American structures that affect pregnant women generally further reinforce the possibility of surrogate as charge and also suggest that there can be a constructive element involved in making a charge function as such. The United States holds the unenviable title of being the developed country with the highest maternal mortality rate, with an upward trend that defies the global one. Whereas global rates fell by approximately 30 percent between 2000 and 2015, the rate in the United States rose approximately 45 percent to 29 deaths per 100,000 women. In contrast, Iran, which had 123 deaths per 100,000 women in 1990, has lowered its death rate 76 percent from 59 to 14 deaths per 100,000 women.[30] The causes of the American rate increase are manifold and complicated: historic underreporting and the rise in maternal age may play a role, as may obesity and diabetes, especially in minority and impoverished populations that often have limited access to health care.[31] Government policies may factor in as well: Medicaid's coverage relates primarily to needs of the baby and not the medical needs of the woman, so while a woman is covered during and immediately after pregnancy, her insurance coverage may drop shortly after the baby's birth, resulting in less follow-up care and complications that can affect mortality either in the short-term aftermath of the birth or in subsequent pregnancies.[32] State policies in Texas that led to the concurrent decline in access to abortion facilities and birth control also played a role in the upsurge in Texas's maternal mortality rate, which is nearly 1.5 times the national average.[33]

Such factors arguably do not come into play in the case of surrogates, who are generally healthy, want to carry a baby, have a track record of low-risk pregnancies, and receive high-quality medical insurance from wealthy intended parents. The rise in unnecessary C-sections, however, can have adverse effects on surrogates, especially during future pregnancies, as C-sections put women at higher risk for placenta accreta, placenta increta, and placenta percreta, life-threatening conditions where the placenta attaches too deeply into the uterine wall and possibly into other organs such as the bladder.[34] The hemorrhaging that can occur with such conditions can be more easily treated if doctors keep hemorrhage kits nearby during birth and delivery, though this is not routine practice across the country.[35]

The United States has a track record of lagging behind its peers in the developed world in regard to maternal health and wellness. Grassroots efforts have generally not focused on maternal health, and the government has been reluctant to step in and implement measures that protect pregnant and postpartum women, whether in the form of state and federal policies that require health care or maternity leave policies that facilitate postpartum recovery, breastfeeding, and postpartum weight loss or that support long-established research on infant attachment. Indeed, one could argue that the United States, as reflected through its legislation, does not value the lives of women as birthers, such that conditions exist that perpetuate high maternal mortality rates and in turn render pregnant women more vulnerable than they need to be. The individuals who collectively construct the culture in the United States therefore become complicit in causing pregnant women to be at higher risk for long-term health consequences and death; these risks could be avoided by bettering maternal health practices. Consequentially, pregnant women in the United States find themselves in a more-subordinate position than pregnancy necessarily requires, causing them to function as charges to a greater extent than they do in other cultures where policies exist that reflect their needs and support them through pregnancy, childbirth, and the postpartum period.

The financial reality of some surrogates may also cause them to function as economic charges even if their health conditions do not. This is paramount in cases where surrogates choose to participate primarily because of their own financial needs since those needs can ground a power dynamic between them and the intended parents in which they are subservient while the intended parents function as economic dependency workers who can provide what the surrogate lacks. The surrogate here needs the intended parents to meet basic economic needs; the intended parent can provide them. But the position of charge that the surrogate adopts also makes her vulnerable because it is so essential for her economic need to be met that exploitation becomes a real possibility.[36]

The Intended Parent as Dependency Worker and Charge

The conditions and treatment of surrogates add complexity to the dependency worker and charge binary because the surrogate takes on the role of dependency worker even as she may fit the role of the charge. Complexity increases further with analysis of intended parents, particularly in regard to the intended mother, who can be situated within both narrower and extended visions of dependency care. As a dependency worker, the intended parent helps meet certain needs of the surrogate as previously delineated. However, the intended parent may also be seen as a charge in both the narrower and extended sense, depending on the interpretation of infertility as either a disability that affects basic needs or one that primarily affects projected desires.

On the one hand, infertile individuals would not find themselves needing the services of a surrogate if they did not desire children, which makes the experience of infertility different from a disability such as Lou Gehrig's disease, where the disorder increasingly impairs function and the ability of the individual to meet basic needs that are necessary for survival, including the ability to eat and maintain personal hygiene. If one treats infertility as a disability, then it is a disability that does not impair basic functions but rather impairs functions that may allow an individual to attain social belonging needs in the desired manner.[37]

What individuals with infertility (taken in isolation from any comorbidities) and an illness like Lou Gehrig's disease share, however, is the inability of certain parts of the body to function according to the societal norm. Many of the dominant cultural standards in the United States are based on the assumption that the individual can walk, eat, and go to the bathroom without assistance. As a result, homes, schools, and other public and private spaces have stairs; museums hang paintings at the eye level of those who walk, not at the eye level of those who are in wheelchairs; restaurants do not provide personal feeders in addition to waiters; and bathrooms do not routinely come with an assistant to help individuals who cannot autonomously use them. Despite changes made as a result of the Americans with Disabilities Act, what did not change is the assumption that the average America is not disabled. The disabled American—and the accommodations made for him or her—remains the exception to the norm, and not the norm itself. Just as societal structures hold as their norm the individual who does not face physical, cognitive, or emotional impairment, so society holds norms around the assumption that adults will have children. American social welfare programs rely on the idea that there will be future generations to pay into them, retirement systems are set up with the assumption that family members—often children—will step in at some level to provide care, and health insurance companies structure costs on the assumption that there will always be a certain number of healthy young people and a certain number of older or infirm individuals. These are but a few instances of programs that depend on the existence of children for their continuation and that reflect the fact that the country values and assumes procreation will occur.[38] Individuals who cannot procreate, then, find themselves unable to achieve the standard society expects and, as a result, find themselves unable to exist within its dominant set of norms and practices, just as those with other forms of disabilities do.

The significance of a given person's infertility may therefore be partially constructed both by society and by the individual so that the culture's expectations of the individual and the individual's desires intersect. This may help explain why one person may encounter little if any emotional reaction to a diagnosis of infertility while another may present symptoms of great distress. In some ways, the hypothetical patient with Lou Gehrig's disease also faces the hurdles of societal construction: were the ALS patient the cultural norm, then the daily life of that individual might look very different than it does in the contemporary United States. Such an individual might have more freedom if everyone spoke with certain movements of their eyes—the eyes do not paralyze during ALS—as opposed to their mouths or if every person received a feeding tube as the normal way of eating. However, even in this hypothetical culture, one might argue that the patient with Lou Gehrig's disease still requires an increasing intensity of physical care as his limbs paralyze: if he cannot stand up or lift a spoon to his mouth, then an external source must help him do so. In contrast, except in situations where infertility is occasioned by other medical conditions such as cancer or endometriosis, infertility in and of itself does not compromise the individual in quite the same way. Put another way, distress for the infertile individual is dependent on the individual's desire for children in a way that distress for the individual with Lou Gehrig's disease—even accounting for social construction—is not. In turn, dependency for the infertile individual predicates itself on that individual's agency in seeking to reproduce. In contrast, the person with Lou Gehrig's disease necessarily finds himself requiring dependency care to meet the basic needs of daily living.[39]

The Significance of Dual Dependencies and Connected Vulnerability

Regardless of the social construction of infertility, what remains is the infertile individual's desire to procreate and inability to do so, placing that individual in a position of dependence on others. The question thus arises of whether surrogacy is unilaterally directed in terms of dependency care—as in the case of other disabilities, where an individual simply cannot reciprocate care due to incapacitation—or whether mutuality and interdependency can factor in. Anthropological research across cultures seems to show that some contexts construct surrogacy with linearity of care directed from surrogate to intended parent, while others present surrogacy with greater mutuality. The surrogate may be said to function as a charge in the latter contexts who needs the intended parents to function as dependency workers to help fulfill her own identity and sense of call; meanwhile, the intended parents undertake the role of charge because they need assistance with procreation. In this setup, there is not only interdependence between charge and dependency worker but also interplay among the individuals holding each role.

The concept of connected vulnerability adds depth to the perspective that surrogates and intended parents can simultaneously position themselves as charge and dependency worker within the dependency dyad, especially if one employs dependency care in its extended sense. Connected vulnerability emerges from absence or negation—something is missing that a person desires to be present. That absence is the absence of offspring in the case of intended parents, whereas for the surrogate, it may be the absence of a financial stability, legacy, belonging, or identity. Recognizing the significance of connected vulnerability in surrogacy requires that one acknowledge that any third-party procedure begins with loss as the starting point, be it the loss of biological parenthood or the loss of ability to fulfill the identity that a person envisioned for him- or herself. Individuals existing in a state of vulnerability may be tempted to invoke protective measures, perhaps by isolating themselves from the community, which in this case might involve creating protective barriers or anonymity in the surrogate-parent relationship. Yet isolation prevents the leap of trust that establishes connection, and without either trust or connection, community cannot materialize.

Acknowledging connected vulnerability in reproduction also discourages the assumption that either members of the family or the family as a unit can exist autonomously. This case might best be made by considering the cases of surrogacy described in India: of the three cultural constructions of surrogacy described in chapter 2, India's construct most privileged surrogacy as a business contract and most downplayed the potential for close relationships between surrogates and intended parents. Dependency care most often appeared as unilateral, directed from the surrogate to the intended parent. As a result, intended parents generally did not have access to the day-to-day lives of surrogates in order to gain an understanding of their experiences, either their joys or their struggles, and it was more acceptable for intended parents to refrain from participating in the process of identity construction with the surrogate or to refrain from a long-term relationship with the surrogate after the baby's birth.[40]

This instantiation of surrogacy signals a unilateral direction of care that appears to correlate with a singular focus of subjectivity, so that the recipient of care remains a subject while the dependency worker takes on the character of an object. In severing connections with the surrogate or by keeping her identity anonymous, for instance, intended parents may be said to objectify the surrogate, relegating her to the status of familial outsider while the child she carried within her womb is not only a familial insider but also—if one assumes that children are a necessary part of families—its catalyst. The contrast between child and surrogate is significant here: as object, the surrogate can be assumed to have fewer rights and privileges in regard to the family than insiders do. It also becomes legitimate to say that the contributions of the surrogate, while necessary and valued in the short term, become immaterial in the long term. As such she is appropriately regarded as an object that rightly belongs outside the family unit, as opposed to a subject who is part of it. In contrast, connected vulnerability acknowledges mutual subjectivity by acknowledging an absence of a self component, whether it be body, desire, agency, or a combination of the three, and by connecting because of this absence, individuals have the possibility to constitute their selves more fully as subjects. The awareness of absence, therefore, creates the possibility of growth. Awareness of vulnerability wrought by self suffering permits mutual self transformation.[41]

The Surrogate and the Family

The current relational dynamics that exist in surrogacy inevitably lead to the question of whether the surrogate ought to be considered part of the family unit, which in turn leads to the question of just what the family is. Proposals that predicate the use of surrogacy on liberal ethics allow for agency but fail to take into account the centrality of relationships to the procedure. Similarly, family definitions rooted in biology not only ignore the role of formative relationships but also fail to consider biblical passages including Mark 1:20, Luke 8:19–21, and Ephesians 1:5, all of which imply that family derives through relational bonds rather than genetic ones. However, even admitting that family ought to be defined by relationship instead of genetics, the question then becomes what kind of relationships should define it. A parent who physically abuses, emotionally harms, or objectifies a child might have a relationship with that child, but it seems counterintuitive to suggest that such forms should be normative for the family or should be imitated by others.

A more expansive utilization of the dependency worker and charge model may be useful in defining the kinds of relationships that characterize the family. This requires something of an expansion of Kittay's scholarship: Kittay discusses scenarios in which dependency work is unidirectional because of the unique needs of the charges involved, and even within her understanding of expanded dependency work, the focus of care is always from dependency worker to charge and not the reverse. As a result, it is the dependency worker who meets the needs of the charge while the charge is unable to meet the needs of the dependency worker. Families, however, are not necessarily set up this way, though at first glance they may appear to be. Consider a two-parent household with a newborn where one parent is on maternity leave to care for the newborn while the other works. The newborn appears to fit the role of the charge, depending on the parents for breastmilk or formula, clothing, diaper changes, and a place to sleep. The parents are physically, emotionally, and financially responsible for the newborn, and the newborn appears to be in no position to meet the needs of the parents. What the newborn does provide, however, is a new identity for the adults in the system, turning them into parents instead of a married childless couple by virtue of the responsibilities that these particular adults have for this particular child. That parental identity is not something they could procure for themselves but rather one that must be procured through the existence of another human being entrusted to their care, such that they are dependent on the child for the creation of it. In this way, the infant directly addresses the desire of each adult to be a parent and transforms the self of the parent into the self that the parent wants to realize. Such care is not mutual (the infant does not provide food or clothing for the parents) nor is it interdependent (again because the infant and parents do not depend on each other in synonymous ways). However, there exists dependence in the form of connected vulnerability across parties because the child requires—and thus is vulnerable to—the parents for physical survival, and the parents require—and thus are vulnerable to—the child for survival of the self. This kind of dependency care might be labeled as consonant. In consonant dependency care, members of the system enhance the qualities necessary for the thriving of the other in such a way that they serve simultaneously as dependency worker and charge.[42]

A family is therefore not just a set of individuals who engage in the quest for social belonging and self construction but ones who do so in a specific way, by participating in consonant dependency care in order to ensure that each member can thrive as a self composed of body, desire, and agency. Spouses vow to love and honor one another, to be loyal across time to the self of the other, and to support one another's bodies in sickness and in health. They thereby engage in coconstruction of spousal identity and consonant dependency care in their responsibilities to each other. Similarly, parents try to give their children a variety of opportunities to strengthen their bodies, discover their desires, and pursue their dreams, while children establish long-desired identities of parents and become the fulfillment of the actions they took to conclude their reproductive story. Each member of the family exists as a particular self because of the role that other members of the family play: as simultaneous dependency workers and charges, these individuals not only provide physical care but also enhance the desires and agency of the individual, connected through unique vulnerabilities and the commitment to consonant dependency care that in turn facilitates social belonging.

Such a definition expands the sphere of who might be considered a member of the family, because while the individuals one lives with may be obvious participants in consonant dependency care, others outside the home may also engage in it. Consider again the hypothetical two-parent household with their single infant. As the infant ages, she craves a sibling, asking her parents repeatedly for a younger brother or sister because she wants a close friend who will always be part of her life; however, the parents are not interested in having any more children. The little girl is also very physically active, so her parents sign her up for soccer, for which she shows a natural propensity, and she immediately develops close relationships with her teammates and deep respect for her coach. Her coach believes in the girl's ability and encourages her to keep developing her skills. The coach stresses the importance of loyalty between the teammates instead of competition, and over time the girl begins to think of her teammates as close friends. The team plays through middle school and high school, and the girl remains close with the members and her coach even after she leaves for college. She becomes a soccer coach after graduation and opens her own gym for young children. Her coach and her teammates attend her wedding and several even serve as bridesmaids; at the reception, the bride publicly remarks that she would not be the adult she is today without the girls on her childhood soccer team and her coach's support. Her teammates and her coach make similar remarks at the reception.

This soccer team would not be considered a family if family were defined either by biology or by residential relationships, but team members could be considered family if one references the trifecta of social belonging, self construction, and consonant dependency care because of the dependence that each individual had on the other, especially in regard to the self. The coach, for instance, felt called to the work of forming an elite team of players; she received payment for this work and may not have undertaken the work without remuneration because she needed some kind of income to pay her rent, but the payment did not detract from the coach's sense that the girls shaped her identity and allowed her to fulfill her sense of call or her dream of being a coach. In this way, the coach needed the girls to fulfill her identity, just as the girls needed the coach to teach them soccer, simultaneously allowing them to serve in consonant dependency worker and charge roles. The girls also functioned similarly among themselves: together they were able to pursue their desires, manifest their dreams, and transform their bodies to perform certain feats, with each offering crucial support to the identity formation of the other. The consonant dependency care extended between the girls, and between girls and coach, therefore united them so each member's self components could thrive, in turn giving them a sense of social belonging and thus making them a family.

If one employs consonant dependency care as the defining factor of the family, then it becomes possible to suggest that the surrogate, intended parents, and resulting child or children are all rightly considered to be a family, provided participants employ surrogacy in a constructive fashion. In other words, the injurious and resistive forms of surrogacy discussed in chapter 3 fail to meet the criteria of consonant dependency care wherein each member functions simultaneously as dependency worker and charge in relation to some component of the self. In constructive surrogacy, however, each participant counters alienation, instead participating in a process that seeks to uphold the body, desire, and agency of all members of the system.

Just because it is possible to instantiate surrogacy in this way does not mean that humans should, and just because it is possible to think of the surrogate as a family member does not necessarily mean it is advisable. However, both practical wisdom and theological tradition advocate for broader family constructions than ones defined either by genetics or by residential address, as reinforced by psychological and anthropological research that suggests the healthiest reproductive relationships emerge from a sense of mutual discernment between individuals rather than from an obligation predetermined by a shared last name or shared DNA. Passages from the Bible complement this perspective: Jesus eschews his biological family in Luke's Gospel, instead stating that all those who adhere to the gospel are his true siblings and parents (Luke 8:19-21); he instructs the Beloved Disciple to treat Mary as his mother during the crucifixion (John 19:25-27); and God images the divine self as parent to children in multiple biblical passages (2 Sam 7:14; 2 Cor 6:18; Gal 4:4-5; Eph 1:5; Rom 8:14). These passages expand the vision of family and, as a consequence, expand the sphere of those with whom we share the task of consonant dependency care.

Conclusion

Imaging the family as a system engaged in consonant dependency care for the purpose of self construction and social belonging recognizes that at various times and in various ways we are all likely to be "the least of these" and find ourselves in need of care (Matt 25:40). Members of the family provide that care in ways that feel most authentic to their sense of self, recognizing that they may receive consonant care either synchronously or asynchronously.

Such a vision not only creates the possibility of viewing the surrogate as a family member; it also creates the possibility of integrating multiple other individuals into the family who might ordinarily be considered to exist outside of it, in turn transforming assumptions about who functions as an insider and who functions as an outsider in a given family system. The implications for this expanded vision of family therefore extend beyond the realm of surrogacy and assisted reproduction and into broader societal conversations about how we structure nonreproductive surrogate relationships and construct their meaning in the United States.

Conclusion

Generalized Surrogacy and a Global Family

Many Americans believe that the family is the basic moral unit of society and that how humans structure relationships inside the family influences how they structure relationships outside of it. Family thereby becomes a locus of relational formation and a relational testing ground so that beliefs and practices developed first within the family extend to beliefs and practices with society at large. What the family is, who belongs in a given unit, and what harm and healing can look like within it therefore may have implications that extend from the single family to a broader collective. As prior chapters argued, kinship ought not to define family; rather, family is a unit of social belonging that utilizes consonant dependency care in order to ensure that each member can thrive as a self composed of body, desire, and agency. Casting aside the primacy of kinship allows for a more expansive vision of family that includes the surrogate as valued member. However, the surrogate is not the only individual who becomes a family member under this new definition: anyone who participates in the process of consonant dependency care for the purpose of mutual self construction has the potential to do so.

Two questions emerge from this assertion. The first is whether individuals beyond reproductive surrogates could be considered non–kinship-based family members. In other words, can individuals become family without being joined by blood, marriage, or other forms of reproduction, including surrogacy or gamete donation? Should, for instance, a child's teacher be considered part of the family? Or what about one's boss or best friend, the mail carrier to whom one never speaks, or the next-door neighbors to whom one does, but only preceding vacations when they need someone to pick up the mail? The possibility that all of these individuals might be considered family members exists given the abovementioned definition, thus leading to the question of whether there are familial boundaries or if we are, in fact, one universal family.

The second question that emerges as a result of the prior conclusions is whether the conception of family proposed in this book is consonant with Christianity. It may be proposing a vision of family that, while salutary, is antithetical to Christianity or unrelated to it. Drawing together previous conclusions provided by the social sciences, Christian theology, and biblical texts in prior chapters will therefore draw together this particular study in practical theology.

The Expansiveness of Family and the Generalized Surrogate

Delores Williams provides an extensive evaluation of surrogacy for the Christian tradition in *Sisters in the Wilderness*, using the Sarah and Hagar story to argue that surrogacy is essentially harmful because it necessarily results in exploitation of the surrogate by those in positions of power.[1] Proceeding to use both historical and contemporary examples from the lives of black women of both literal and symbolic—what she calls "social-role"—surrogacy, Williams argues that there can be nothing redemptive, even positive, in surrogate experiences because of their essentially exploitative nature. However, while Williams' conclusions can be a compelling interpretation of surrogacy when evaluated from the perspective of black women's lives or, more expansively, from the perspective of the life of any individual who exists in a position of systemic or individual subordination, this study has proposed that perhaps Williams' conclusions cannot be universally applied, and that instead of surrogacy being essentially negative, surrogacy's negativity predicates itself upon the power dynamics that situate it as well as the value that each member of the surrogacy arrangement places upon the self construction of the other. The conditions, then, for healthy surrogacy most appropriately originate from a desire for mutual self construction rather than exploitation or objectification. This fashions surrogacy, at its best, into a vocation.

What Williams and this work share, however, is a realization that surrogacy extends beyond the reproductive realm, and thus the same risks and benefits that apply to reproductive surrogacy extend to nonreproductive surrogacy. The term *surrogate*, at its broadest, means a proxy, someone who substitutes for another in a given service or role. Surrogacy therefore calls on one person—Person A—to complete a task for Person B that is important to Person B's self-preservation or self-actualization. Examples of this kind of generalized surrogacy are available in multitudinous contexts in the United States. From a historical perspective, Williams identifies instances where black women served as mammies or instances where they were raped in order to provide pleasure for the slaveholder while protecting a white wife's role as a sexual partner for procreative purposes only.[2] The examples Williams provides of social-role surrogacy are coercive, and appropriate to the context to which she writes, but one could also identify examples that potentially, at least, lack this coercive element: butchers pluck and slaughter chickens, allowing a woman to fulfill her dream of being a stay-at-home mother who can pick up dinner at the grocery store instead of having to slaughter the chicken herself; factory workers manufacture telephones with video capability so a recent college graduate can take a job overseas but still maintain a visual relationship with the partner he wants to marry; daycare workers provide a nurturing environment and educational opportunities to young children so their parents can meet their professional and economic goals; a cardiologist assesses the heart health of a patient so that the patient does not to cull the information or run tests himself; one friend drives another to the airport when that individual's car breaks down so he can make his flight; one member of Alcoholics Anonymous sponsors a newcomer who seeks sobriety; a writer publishes a book of fiction that a retiree purchases in order to escape the monotony of her daily routine.[3] The body of Person A substitutes for the body of Person B in each of these cases so that Person B can exercise agency toward multiple desires simultaneously—the one that Person B uses his or her own body for and the one that Person B uses the body of Person A for. Person B is thus the obvious receiver of goods and benefits in nonreproductive surrogacy, while Person A's role is far more nebulous, dependent on how Person B engages Person A. The two types of generalized surrogacy outlined below therefore hinge upon the treatment and benefits afforded to Person A.

The Self of Person A in Self-Defeating Generalized Surrogacy

Self-defeating surrogacy permits a hierarchy of selves that situates the needs of the self of one participant (Person B) above those of another so that the kind of domination exerted upon the surrogate, Person A, in any form of self-defeating surrogacy harms, or at least does not enhance, the self. This would be the type of surrogacy Williams describes in *Sisters in the Wilderness*. A question arises, however, as to whether the self of Person B really does benefit in the end from self-defeating surrogacy, and whether there is a distinction between perceived and actual benefits. Consider, for example, an adult male in California who consumes meat on a daily basis—meat that is slaughtered by nonunionized immigrant workers living in Iowa and that originates in a facility that restricts the movement and diet of animals in order to manufacture most efficiently the inexpensive meat desired by adult men. The immigrant workers make below minimum wage, work overtime without proper compensation, receive no health-care or retirement benefits, and engage regularly in physically dangerous work practices. Several of their colleagues have sustained injuries on the job that rendered them disabled. One factory worker, for example, also dreamed of being a musician in his home country but came to the United States illegally after his wife became pregnant in order to secure greater financial stability for his family.

This benefit to the self perceived by the factory worker—Person A—is problematic in this scenario. The worker has employment, which may sustain the basic needs of the body, but the type and terms of that employment are far from ideal. Even if one argued that the worker enhanced the bodily component of the self, it is hard to see how either desire or agency sustain or enhance; the worker's self does not benefit from this generalized surrogacy arrangement.

In contrast, the Californian carnivore in this scenario functions as Person B who uses the immigrant factory worker as a surrogate in order to procure the meat he desires without having to raise and slaughter it himself. The meat eater benefits, from his point of view, because he attains the product he wants at the price he wants it and sustains his body with the calories he seeks on the terms that he desires. However, the question here is whether his perception alone is a sufficiently substantive reason to say that his self actually benefits from the arrangement.

A return to earlier discussions of corporate sin as cultural misorientation may be of use here. Chapter 3 argued that cultural misorientation affects intended parents insofar as overarching structures in society limit the freedom of intended parents to make and enact reproductive decisions. The same may be said for generalized surrogacy: cultural misorientation limits the freedom and the viewpoints of individuals who engage in generalized surrogacy so that the fullness of what is at stake in a given surrogate procedure for the self of involved parties may not be easily discernable because of overarching discourses, power structures, and worldviews that exist beyond the individual. In the example above, for instance, the meat consumer might have no knowledge of the factory worker's reality because he has not been exposed to the conditions of a meatpacking plant and did not seek them out. Both of these reasons may say something about Person B as an individual, but they may also reflect what Person B inherited through cultural misorientation: individualism, geographical distance, lack of documentation or publicity about harm, are just some potential forms of cultural misorientation that could cause him to be predisposed not to investigate the conditions of the factory worker. As a result, the self of Person B participates—either willingly or through omission—in the cultural misorientation that harms Person A.[4] Self-defeating surrogacy, then, shares much with injurious surrogacy because each cultural misorientation negatively affects each party in a way that prevents all parties from growing and thriving. In addition, each turns the surrogate into a scapegoat for the purpose of privileging the self of Person B.

The power relations that exist between parties in self-defeating generalized surrogacy could be extended to those seen in larger-scale societal problems so that one might be able to read these issues in terms of generalized surrogate relationships. Ageism is a phenomenon wherein those who are part of one age group (Group B) disregard the selves of those who are part of another (Group A) in order to validate their own bodies' superiority. Racism allows people of one skin color (Group B) to deem themselves superior to people of another skin color (Group A) so that they can maintain power across societal contours and thereby have greater ease when it comes to meeting their own needs, whether they relate to body, desire, or agency. Sexism functions much the same way, only this time it is the sexed body that justifies access to cultural power. The acceptance of policies that perpetuate poverty allows those with financial resources (Group B) to see themselves as harder workers or morally superior to those without them (Group A). The high incarceration and recidivism rates among certain groups in the United States likewise allow those who exist outside of the prison system a sense of self-superiority at the expense of those who exist inside of it.[5] Rape and sexual assault can be read as events in which perpetrators objectify the victim's self in order to manifest their perceptions of their own power or fulfill their own sexual pleasure.[6] In all of these cases, Group B needs Group A in order to enhance its desired self-concept, so that Group A functions as the surrogate who meets the perceived needs of Group B. Meanwhile, Group B achieves those perceived needs at the expense of Group A, essentially scapegoating Group A to do so and robbing Group A of the opportunity to sustain or enhance the self. Each of these scenarios also emerges from connected vulnerability gone awry—Group B harms Group A because Group B perceives a self vulnerability. But instead of using that vulnerability to foster mutual connection and growth, Group B uses its power to exploit Group A because it believes that so doing will strengthen its perceived weaknesses. At its worst, then, generalized surrogacy permits abuses of power by one person or group toward another, validating exploitation, perpetuating vulnerability, and creating structures that permit the belief that some selves are worth more than others.

The Role of Power in Self-Defeating Generalized Surrogacy

Self-defeating generalized surrogacy harms or eradicates the subjectivity of at least one participant in the surrogacy relationship so that the self experiences not enhancement but defeat through harm done to body, desire, agency, or a combination of the three. It most clearly involves harm to the individual serving as a proxy for another individual who desires the proxy for self-preservation or self-actualization, though self-defeating surrogacy could also involve injury to both parties.

The function of power proves pivotal to understanding how self-defeating generalized surrogacy operates as well as to understanding the distinction between self-defeating and self-enhancing surrogacy. Consider power in terms of two categories: the ability to exert power over another ("power-over") and the ability to exert power in order to accomplish something ("power-to-do").[7] Power-to-do is present in both forms of generalized surrogacy, insofar as Person B desires to—and subsequently does—exert agential power to engage a proxy who can preserve or enhance his or her self. In multiple-self-enhancing surrogacy, Person B also uses power-to-do as proxy to preserve or enhance the self of Person A and Person A does the reverse. In contrast, power-over plays a definitive role in self-defeating surrogacy, with Person B wielding power-to-do by enacting agency as power-over Person A in such a way that Person A enhances or preserves the self of Person B while being unable to exert power-to-do. As a result, Person A's subjectivity suffers.[8] The distinction between multiple-self-enhancing and self-defeating surrogacy could thereby be explained through reference to the idea that power-over functions as domination that situates the body, desire, and agency of one party above that of the other, while power-to-do functions as mutual empowerment that benefits the self components of both.

Multiple-Self-Enhancing Generalized Surrogacy

If self-defeating generalized surrogacy echoes the dynamics Williams describes in her exploration of black women's experiences of surrogacy, highlighting the potentially coercive nature of surrogacy, then multiple-self-enhancing generalized surrogacy may be defined as a surrogacy arrangement that lacks this coercive element. This form benefits the selves of both Person A and Person B, either inside or outside the reproductive sphere. Although Person B's needs might immediately motivate the need for a surrogate, Person A retains subjectivity, much as in constructive reproductive surrogacy, where each individual participates out of desire and is able to exercise agency toward attaining that desire through surrogacy, or in consonant dependency care, where each member affects the other's self development in a positive way. Consonant dependency care and constructive surrogacy can therefore be considered examples of multiple-self-enhancing generalized surrogacy, but examples certainly extend beyond the reproductive realm. Teacher-student relationships, romantic relationships, parent-child relationships, sibling relationships, work-based relationships, and friendships all have the capacity to function this way, as do other relationships. Friendship, in particular, be a paradigmatic form of multiple-self-enhancing surrogacy because the nonhierarchical potential of the relationship could make it easier for participants to enact mutual power-to-do.

Social-Identity Support in Friendship as Multiple-Self-Enhancing Generalized Surrogacy

Friendship is a commitment between two individuals rooted in proximity, mutual intimacy, and mutual self construction involving one party upholding the root desired identity of another as it relates to a particular group or set of characteristics so that the individual is able to more fully inhabit that self. Proximity therefore allows for the initial creation of friendships,[9] while mutual intimacy ensures a level of reciprocity in terms of personal self-disclosure. It is less likely for Zach, say, to become friends with Kelly if Zach talks incessantly and shares every detail of his life but expresses no interest in the life of Kelly than it is if both parties agree on and reciprocate self-disclosure. It is also not the utility that Kelly provides to Zach that results in friendship, because it is not the exchange of concrete goods that grounds their friendship in mutual intimacy but rather a shared commitment to gaining familiarity with and responding to the self-development needs of the other.[10]

Social-identity support further grounds the friendship that proximity and mutual intimacy initiate, yet social-identity support requires that one be able to identify with something as a reference point for self construction. The existence of groups and group identification becomes pivotal in this regard. If an individual—this time named Kevin—desires strength, flexibility, and discipline, and sees these qualities as essential to his future self, then he may join a karate club where he can not only practice these skills but also receive positive reinforcement concerning them from other members of the group. Kevin therefore takes steps to construct his own sense of self by joining and participating in a group that matches his root desires, just as his self-concept also receives reinforcement through the friendships he has with others who identify him as a martial artist.[11]

Research on close friendships suggests that "best friends" often share membership in the same group because it enables social-identity support; however, best friends are also likely to participate in different groups and remain affirmative of one another's roles in their respective memberships. So sameness is not the prerequisite for friendship; rather, a willingness to support the unique future self that a given individual seeks to inhabit is. To that end, two future friends—here called Jill and Jane—might meet in a college English class that the school requires for graduation. Jill wants to be a rabbi; Jane wants to be a human rights lawyer. Jill and Jane do not share a love of English literature—they both take the class because of the college's requirement—and the class does not directly offer them social-identity support. Instead, the class provides an opportunity for them to get to know one another. By the end of the semester, Jill talks with her parents about her "lawyer" friend and Jane talks with her roommate about her "rabbi" friend, and each person delights in the self the other seeks. To mutually support those future selves, Jill reads Jane's law school application, Jane attends Jill's graduation from rabbinic school, and each asks regularly how the other is doing in relation to the achievement of her respective goals. Jill and Jane therefore reinforce the other's membership in a given group—for Jill, a group of rabbis, and for Jane, a group of lawyers—though neither participates in the other's group affiliation.[12]

Social-identity support therefore functions as a form of reciprocity within friendship that specifically relates to the formation and maintenance of self-concept. This reciprocity does not equate to sameness, but it does result in what might be considered an equal benefit to each party because that benefit is the one desired by each party. It therefore mirrors the kind of reciprocity seen in constructive surrogacy, where the surrogate helps intended parents achieve their identity as caregivers while intended parents help the surrogate achieve her identity goals, perhaps as a social hero. Neither participates in the same group or has the same goal for the self; however, each is able to support the cultivation of the other's desired self through shared participation in reproduction. Subjectivity of Person A and Person B is therefore maintained in constructive surrogacy much as it is maintained in cases where social-identity support culminates in close friendships.[13]

One might query whether the kind of identity construction that constitutes friendship is necessarily salutary. A person could desire, for instance, to become a Nazi leader or an ISIS martyr or a serial killer, such that an individual's desired self was prima facie morally reprehensible. Similarly, a woman could dream of becoming George Clooney's wife and ask her best friend to help disrupt his marriage to Amal Clooney in order to achieve that end. Such an outcome might benefit the woman, but it would certainly harm Amal. Finally, a woman might seek to become a porn star who regularly participates in bondage, sadomasochism, or coercive sexual activity, but if the videos she records cause the men who watch them to treat abusive sexual behaviors as the norm, then her chosen self exponentially harms women.

Such examples do not constitute true friendship, because friendship is not predicated upon one person coconstructing the identity of another without limitation. In each of the preceding scenarios, the person who supports the particular desires of the individuals may be said to be more of an enabler than a friend. If the desired self does not uphold the body, desires, or agency of others beyond just the individual in question, then what is expressed may be said to be a negative projected desire and not a root.[14] Friends at their best, therefore, not only support others in their quest for self construction but also name and challenge misplaced constructive goals. The extent to which a friend can see the distinction may well rest on the power of cultural misorientation, though, efficacy aside, such responsibility to name and help transform misplaced constructive aims remains the goal.

Positive Characteristics of Multiple-Self-Enhancing Generalized Surrogacy

Friendship provides one concrete example of multiple-self-enhancing generalized surrogacy; constructive surrogacy and consonant dependency care provide others. What each shares is a commitment to mutual self construction occasioned by the need for each party to serve as a proxy for the other in regard to a given role or service that the individual cannot autonomously complete. An individual needs another human to function as a friend in order to be a friend and vice versa; a parent needs a younger human being to function as a child, and a child needs an adult to function as a parent; a student needs someone with a certain body of knowledge to teach her chemistry and a teacher needs someone who does not have that body of knowledge to function as a student who wants to learn it. Each of these potentially could become instantiations of multiple-self-enhancing surrogacy because each engages multiple participants as proxies for self-deficits that the other can fill.

However, the mere presence of the proxy is not enough for a relationship to fit the definition of multiple-self-enhancing generalized surrogacy. Consider sibling relationships as an example: a set of heterosexual parents biologically birth two children. Those children seem to have a relationship like Cane and Abel's from the start, each hurling insults at the other, engaging in regular physical combat, and stating that they wish they did not live in the same house. They grow estranged as soon as they do not live in the same residence and never speak again. Consider a different hypothetical set of siblings, both adopted. This set of siblings gets along well, considers the other to be a best friend, joyously attends the other's artistic performances or sporting events and every graduation. As adults, they serve as each other's maid of honor or best man and become a treasured aunt or uncle to the other sibling's children. Each describes the other as a great gift and says that life would not be the same—indeed, it would be emptier and far less enjoyable—without the sibling.

A cursory contrast of these two instantiations of siblinghood reveals one relationship that may broadly be characterized as broken and another that may broadly be characterized as loving. In each configuration of siblinghood, Sibling A is required in order for Sibling B to be a sibling and vice versa (one cannot, in other words, identify as a sibling autonomously, in isolation from all other human beings). However, there is a qualitative difference between the first hypothetical example and the second that cannot be explained by shared genes, because the non-genetically related siblings possess a healthier relationship than the biologically related ones. And while one might object with reference to the hypothetical nature of this example, only a cursory observation of real-life sibling relationships reveals that biology alone does not determine the quality of the relationship. Parental favoritism, age gaps, gender, poor communication among family members, and differences in values can all lead to either close or distanced sibling relationships. As a result, the health of sibling relationships is not determined by the biological connection or even that there is a biological connection between one sibling and another; rather, the overall health of sibling relationships depends on the way one self engages the other.

In sum, then, while Sibling A exists as a surrogate that makes Sibling B into a sibling and vice versa, it is the quality of the relationship between the siblings that determines the quality of the surrogacy and whether it functions as multiple-self-enhancing or -defeating. If both siblings validate the desired future self of the other and help to coconstruct it, then such siblinghood might be multiple-self-enhancing. However, if one denies the subjectivity of the other or seeks to annihilate or dictate its parameters, then mutual self construction does not occur and there is no reciprocal self enhancement or growth. Such instances, then, would not rightly be considered self-enhancing generalized surrogacy but instead might more appropriately be situated under the category of self-defeating generalized surrogacy.

The Significance of Generalized Surrogacy

The two types of generalized surrogacy outlined above assert that healthy surrogacy practices must maintain the selves of all participants. This in and of itself, however, does not mean that what they are doing constitutes family. In the case of self-defeating surrogacy, affronts to the self certainly do not mirror the kind of consonant dependency care that defines family. However, when participants practice multiple-self–enhancing generalized surrogacy, then the reverse appears to be true.

Consequently, if it is indeed the case that surrogacy extends beyond reproduction, and if it is true that surrogates, because of their role in constructing identity, can be, in ideal circumstances, considered part of the family, then the consequence is that family is far broader than what a definition predicated on biological kinship allows us to conceive. It means that members of our community at large are not only teachers, coworkers, service providers, or friends. They are family. Indeed, it is likely that even strangers ought to be considered part of the family because of the role that they potentially play in identity construction and social belonging. As a result, it becomes incumbent upon each individual to recognize that one who seems foreign is be acknowledged and welcomed as family. In other words, it is not simply that we are each in this life together; it is that we *are* together because of the way that each of us cocreates the life of another. To act otherwise is to act in a way that self-defeats.

Additionally, it is not just that the sphere of who is considered family widens beyond initial conception. It is that surrogates are more important than one might think. Each of us needs surrogates. We need them not just to birth children but to birth ourselves. Likewise, each of us is a surrogate insofar as we participate in the metaphorical birth of other selves. Our communities depend upon the existence of surrogates for their health such that the community's well-being predicates itself on whether individual members operate in ways that are self-defeating or mutually self-enhancing. A society with wealth inequality, for instance, might be said to be founded upon principles that support self-defeating surrogacy, where those with little become surrogates for those with much, because they are coerced into positions of inequality and take on the burdens of poverty so that wealthy individuals can inhabit the identity they crave.

It therefore becomes incumbent upon us to name the universality of family and, in turn, to create structures that support multiple-self-enhancing surrogacy both inside and outside the reproductive sphere. Indeed, it may be especially important to implement such expansiveness within the reproductive sphere because this may provide the most fertile ground—pun intended—for practicing these kinds of expansive familial relationships and then translating them to the context of the wider world. Such practice may take multitudinous forms that include, but are not limited to, employing a reproductive surrogate, understanding friends to be as valuable as biological relatives, teaching one's children that blood matters less than relationship, and treating those outside the biological family—even strangers—with the same kindness, respect, and generosity as those within it. Once again, therefore, it becomes necessary to challenge those structures that reinforce the primacy of the nuclear biological family, that create a culture of familial insiders and outsiders, that predicate themselves upon hierarchy and power inequalities, in order to open the possibility for wider, deeper relationships as well as greater accountability.

What Makes This Practical Theology of Family "Christian"

Jesus' life and the ensuing New Testament writings that emerged from it reflect a vision of family extending beyond biological lines: Jesus tells Mary and the Beloved Disciple from the cross to treat one another as mother and son (John 19:25-27); he proclaims that his true mother and brothers were those who followed the word of God (Luke 8:21).[15] Baptism and the Eucharist also both reconfigure relationships so that the baptized individual becomes a member of the family of believers while the Eucharist unites followers to Christ by his blood.[16] Christianity's non-biologically based image of family also resonates with Jesus' own familial structure: born to a virgin and raised as a son by a father who was displaced in the reproductive process by the Holy Spirit, one might consider Jesus' own birth to be an early instance of third-party-assisted reproduction—though the Bible does not specify the genetic makeup of Jesus' DNA to validate this claim.

This book's assertion that biology alone does not define the family is therefore nothing new to Christianity. However, reclaiming the language of surrogacy in relation to understanding family is. The surrogate—literal or symbolic—is necessary to the construction of the self, essential to the fulfillment of body, desire, and agency. Put differently, the surrogate is crucially important to creation itself, the acknowledgment of which elevates the role, provided that the surrogate is not participating because of coercion or self-defeating mechanisms. Such an assertion also contextualizes New Testament claims that those who do the will of God become brothers and sisters to one another in a way that displaces biology as the primary determinant of those titles, and it insists that this non-biologically based brotherhood and sisterhood is made possible by those who serve in surrogate roles. For if God's will is for human flourishing, and if surrogates facilitate that, then surrogacy, at its best, manifests that kind of flourishing God wishes for humanity.

Generalized Surrogates as Bringers of Hope

At stake here is a reclaiming of the importance of surrogacy that removes the emphasis upon sacrifice and places it instead in conversation with the many instances where God fulfills the promise of hope in response to suffering. Here it is worthwhile to return to chapters 1 and 2, which provided evidence to support the claim that reproductive surrogates often become the embodiment of hope for those who experience infertility and reproductive loss. They help individuals rewrite the ending to a reproductive story that seems impossible to write, allowing those individuals to restore a sense of agency in the process. Reproductive surrogates are also an embodied response to the tough questions that traumas bring about—questions like "Why me?" and "What now?"—and thereby craft meaning in their aftermath. Indeed, insofar as infertility or reproductive loss can be framed in terms of theodicy, one could surmise that reproductive surrogates are women who can address this particular problem of evil directly.[17]

This is what generalized surrogates do as well: in self-enhancing surrogacy, men and women function as individuals who offer the best of humanity to another through their ability to support and coconstruct the self. But the task these generalized surrogates undertake is not without reciprocity, for it is the recipient who does similar work in kind. At its best, then, the generalized surrogate has the potential to address many forms of suffering with the gift of relationship. Indeed, healing from trauma in any form requires connection and meaning-making, two things that the generalized surrogate is uniquely situated to address as coconstructor of the self.[18] The friend who believes the story of a rape survivor, the therapist who counsels the flood victim, or the foster parent who adopts an abused child all function as generalized surrogates who offer the gift of self reconnection.

This image of family as a universal set of hope bringers complements Christianity's own belief that relationship defeats evil, that covenant promises are promises of the transformative power wrought through relationships.[19] Surrogacy, when done well, therefore symbolizes one of the most elegant assurances of Christianity—namely, that which vows that God, through relationship, gifts transformation. What humans do among themselves as coconstructing surrogates thereby imitates the kind of relationship God has with humans.

The Self and Community in Generalized Surrogacy

If generalized surrogacy is ever permissible, the conditions under which it occurs must be ones in which the self of both parties can attempt to flourish in relation to their trifold components of body, desire, and agency. These conditions are not just generated by the individuals involved in a given surrogacy instantiation; rather, they are conditions that emerge from communal structures, from the laws, norms, beliefs, and discourses that define a given culture. It is ultimately the culture's health, then, that affects the potential health of individual surrogacy arrangements, be they reproductive or generalized. As long as cultural misorientation maintains its grip, surrogacy will bear its impression, and until that grip loosens, surrogacy will not be free.[20]

It may be tempting, in light of these conclusions, to discard surrogacy entirely and to argue that there is no scenario in which surrogacy does not function in an injurious or self-defeating way. This interpretation sacrifices the potential that self-enhancing or constructive surrogacy has for giving individuals or groups the opportunity to offer the best they can offer in the simultaneous service of love of neighbor and love of self. Far from being sacrificial, these salutary forms of surrogacy allow humans to grow in their own charisms while also enabling others to do the same, so that each person thrives because their relationships strengthen each self through connected vulnerability. This kind of being is the best of what one human can offer another—the chance to grow, the chance to transform. It is a great gift, and yet it is also given in the hope that one's own self receives the gift in kind so that mutual growth emerges and injurious relationships cease.

Conclusion

Suffering leads to vulnerability, and vulnerability leads to a desire for something beyond it, with the individual standing at a crossroads destined either for further suffering and harm or for community of a type that can cofacilitate a given self's healing process. Individuals at the crossroads must decide which path to take, a choice that might be informed or determined by external influences such as cultural misorientation. Insofar as reproductive surrogacy is concerned, these values affect a given person's framework for contracting with a surrogate and for structuring the surrogate relationship in certain ways; parallel generalized surrogacy dynamics exist outside the reproductive sphere, seeking the same ends.

Surrogacy at its best therefore allows a person to offer a part of him- or herself to enhance the self of another and to receive self benefits in kind. Surrogacy at its worst exploits vulnerabilities and harms the self of participants through abuses of power that seem to put the worst of humanity on display. Yet to discard surrogacy—be it reproductive or generalized—is to cast aside the possibility that humanity can be at its finest when it seeks to create new life, be it new life in the form of personal transformation or new life in the form of a baby whose body, cold, crying, naked, and vulnerable, emerges into the world, incapable of surviving without others who will coconstruct her self, even as, in her nascent state, she may do likewise.

Notes

Introduction

1 "Infertility," Centers for Disease Control and Prevention, July 15, 2016, https://www.cdc.gov/nchs/fastats/infertility.htm.

2 Though the context and content differ, James Gilligan makes a similar argument about small systems within society representing the overarching beliefs and power structures of society at large when he writes about the American prison system. For more on his view that the prison functions as a metaphor of societal beliefs and power, see James Gilligan, *Violence: Reflections on a National Epidemic* (New York: Vintage Books, 1997).

3 Don Browning argues that practice and theory are so integrally intertwined that one does not exist in isolation from the other; all practices are theory laden and all theories are rooted in practice. Similarly, Miroslav Volf argues that practices shape beliefs while beliefs shape practices; ergo, practices can lead to a deeper embrace of belief. Meanwhile, Kathryn Tanner argues that theological reflection is required to ground practices that might otherwise become "slippery" in their meaning and affiliation with Christianity; hence, theory-laden practices always necessitate theological inquiry as a kind of system of checks and balances. See Don Browning, *A Fundamental Practical Theology: Descriptive and Strategic Proposal* (Minneapolis: Fortress, 1991), 6; Miroslav Volf, "Theology for a Way of Life," in *Practicing Theology: Beliefs and Practices in Christian Life*, ed. Miroslav Volf and Dorothy C. Bass (Grand Rapids: Eerdmans, 2002), 250–51; and Kathryn Tanner, "Theological Reflection and Christian Practices," in Volf and Bass, *Practicing Theology*, 234, 239.

4 Poling and Miller refer to this as the process of "critical and constructive reflection within a living community about human experience and interaction." In contrast, Swinton and Mowat refer to this as the "current praxis stage." See James N. Poling and Donald E. Miller, *Foundations for a Practical Theology of Ministry*

(Nashville: Abingdon, 1985), 62; and John Swinton and Harriet Mowat, *Practical Theology and Qualitative Research Methods* (London: SCM Press, 2006), 95.

5 Poling and Miller delineate six types of correlation practical theologians may employ. They define the critical correlational stance as one that involves "insights from the tradition with theories of development and virtue from the human sciences." This book employs such a correlative method. Poling and Miller, *Foundations for a Practical Theology of Ministry*, 47–48.

6 Here I use the term *correlation* to refer to what Poling and Miller term the critical correlational method between the Christian story and social scientific research, which denotes a specific kind of relationship between the Christian story and other perspectives, namely, to take a page from Ogletree, that the Christian story gives meaning to the world by describing God's intentions for it, while social scientific research offers a vocabulary through which to understand the actions of humans in the world. The Christian story therefore imparts meaning to these actions while data concerning the actions—offered by the social sciences—deepens our understanding of God's intentions for the world and the meaning and purpose of it. Thomas Ogletree, "Dimensions of Practical Theology: Meaning, Action, Self," in *Practical Theology: The Emerging Field in Theology, Church, and World* (New York: Harper & Row, 1982), 86.

7 Or, in Don Browning's language, the book moves from "present theory-laden practice to a retrieval of normative theory-laden practice to the creation of more critically held theory-laden practices." *Fundamental Practical Theology*, 5–6.

8 Aaron D. Levine. "Self-Regulation, Compensation, and the Ethical Recruitment of Oocyte Donors," *Hastings Center Report* 40, no. 2 (2010): 25–36.

9 Katie O'Reilly, "When Parents and Surrogates Disagree on Abortion," *The Atlantic*, February 18, 2016.

10 Germany maintains some of the strictest laws concerning assisted reproduction. As Lauren Jade Martin documents, "Germany permits in vitro fertilization and artificial insemination but forbids egg donation, embryo donation, and surrogacy; it also limits the number of embryos that may be transferred to a woman's uterus, forbids sex selection with the exception of cases in which severe sex-linked genetic illness is to be prevented, and forbids unmarried or lesbian women access to assisted reproduction services." Lauren Jade Martin, *Reproductive Tourism in the United States: Creating Family in the Mother Country* (New York: Routledge, 2015), 31. See also S. Bergmann, "Reproductive Agency and Projects: Germans Searching for Egg Donation in Spain and the Czech Republic," *Reproductive BioMedicine Online* 23, no. 5 (November 2011): 600–608.

11 See chapter 2 on Delores Williams for more on Indian medical tourism. See also "Surrogacy as an Infertility Treatment," Fertility Treatment Abroad, http://fertility.treatmentabroad.com/treatments/surrogacy, accessed October 13, 2016.

12 Laws vary concerning surrogacy. The District of Columbia, Louisiana, Michigan, New Jersey, New York, and Washington outlaw the practice entirely. Legal hurdles to using a surrogate also exist in Alaska, Arizona, Iowa, Idaho, Indiana, Missouri, Montana, Nebraska, Tennessee, Virginia, and Wyoming. The remaining states permit surrogacy with limited legal involvement from the

state. See U.S. Surrogacy Law Map, http://www.creativefamilyconnections.com/us-surrogacy-law-map, accessed October 11, 2016.

13 Congregation for the Doctrine of the Faith, *Donum vitae:* Instruction on Respect for Human Life. February 22, 1987, http://www.vatican.va/roman_curia/congregations/cfaith/documents/rc_con_cfaith_doc_19870222_respect-for-human-life_en.html; Congregation for the Doctrine of the Faith, "Instruction *Dignitas personae* on Certain Bioethical Questions," September 8, 2008, http://www.vatican.va/roman_curia/congregations/cfaith/documents/rc_con_cfaith_doc_20081208_dignitas-personae_en.html.

14 Judith Jarvis Thomson, "A Defense of Abortion," *Philosophy and Public Affairs* 1, no. 1 (1971): 47–66.

15 The difference in meaning that a person affords a given reproductive event illustrates that the penning of the reproductive narrative is a process that individuals may use that results in the construction of life itself: the individual who aborts at nine weeks may state that she "aborted a fetus," whereas the woman who miscarries at nine weeks may state that she "lost a baby." The latter woman constructs the loss as a loss of life whereas the other may integrate it into her life's reproductive narrative by affording it a different kind of significance. One may suggest that *fetus* and *baby* are linguistically interchangeable here, yet this may be a reductionistic approach. The woman who aborts may use the term "fetus" precisely because believes she terminated the potential for a life as opposed to a fully formed one, while the woman who miscarried may instead understand herself to have lost a baby to whom she is a mother. The linguistic differences therefore point to significant differences in each woman's interpretation, even though objectively the maturation of both developing humans at nine weeks is the same. One can therefore propose that the difference in these two interpretations derives from how the women write their reproductive narrative and signifies the way that individuals may attempt to construct life itself via linguistic tools in order to form meaning.

1 Infertility, Reproductive Loss, and the Significance of the Biological Family to the Self

1 This biblical text has a long and varied history of interpretation. Augustine held that humanness inhered in the mind so that the mind became the locus of the image of God. In contrast, Irenaeus held that one was born in the image of God but grew, through experiences that yielded wisdom, into the likeness of God. These are two of many patristic interpretations that theologians proposed over millennia. Regardless of the specific pragmatics of what "image" and "likeness" mean, however, theologians tend to agree that humans share in it and thereby share certain divine characteristics. See Alister E. McGrath, *Historical Theology: An Introduction to the History of Christian Thought* (Oxford: Wiley-Blackwell, 1998).

2 To draw the argument further, one could argue that the invocation to be fruitful and multiply is not just a command but also a blessing. See Candida R.

Moss and Joel S. Baden, *Reconceiving Infertility: Biblical Perspectives on Procreation and Childlessness* (Princeton, N.J.: Princeton University Press, 2015), 71.

3 Intriguingly, while the Bible at times frames infertility as a curse, God not only rewards these women with children but then also exalts them, as in the cases of Sarah, Hannah, and Elizabeth. For more context, Moss and Baden present a compelling alternative to this reading that frames barrenness in terms of blessing rather than curse. See Moss and Baden, *Reconceiving Infertility,* 72.

4 Even if one accepts reproduction and children as blessings, a distinction remains between describing procreation as an act that blesses humans or that humans should undertake—claims that still allow for the possibility of intrinsic value apart from reproductive capability—and describing reproduction as the basis for valuing human life. The latter statement imposes instrumental value, supposing that the end a person achieves through the reproductive process justifies his or her existence. Adopting such a stand leads to counterintuitive conclusions, including the possibility that infants and children who are not yet developed enough to reproduce and postmenopausal women who did not bear children are not fully human.

5 Science compounds the conundrum, adding that reproduction is one of the seven characteristics necessary for living beings (the others being environmental responsiveness, the ability to grow and change, the possession of at least one cell, the ability to breathe and possess a metabolism, the ability to maintain homeostasis, and the capability to pass traits to offspring). That said, these criteria primarily refer to what is needed for a species at large to be considered living and not for the individual. The question then arises of which criteria are necessary for a given individual within the species to be considered alive. If an argument can be made that all seven must be present, then the argument can theoretically be made that an individual human being must be able to reproduce in order to be considered alive.

6 The root desires outlined here roughly correlate with Abraham Maslow's hierarchy of needs. Maslow ranked the needs via a pyramid, with physiological needs listed as most primary and self-actualization or self-transcendence listed as most advanced, something to which the individual ascended over time. (Maslow added self-transcendence after originally postulating self-actualization to be the highest-ranking need.) Wahba and Bridwell are among critics who argue that Maslow's hierarchical ranking proves problematic, primarily in that little evidence exists that one must progress from the bottom level of the pyramid in order to reach the top. Correspondingly, root desire does not attempt to rank these needs, arguing only that each is desirable in a fundamental way to individual self-flourishing. See Abraham Maslow, *The Hierarchy of Needs* (Corby, U.K.: Institute of Management Foundation, 1998). See also Mahmoud A. Wahba and Lawrence G. Bridwell, "Maslow Reconsidered: A Review of Research on the Need Hierarchy Theory," *Organizational Behavior and Human Performance* 15, no. 2 (1976): 212–40.

7 One might argue that this is a very Western, individualistic construction of desire, as Geert Hofstede does in his criticism of Maslow's needs-ranking system, arguing that Maslow privileges individualistic over collectivist societies. In contrast to Maslow, however, this proposal about desire does not rank needs hierarchically but rather horizontally, with each need being essential to the individual's self but with none of necessity ranking above or below the others. See Geert Hofstede, "The Cultural Relativity of the Quality of Life Concept," *Academy of Management Review* 9, no. 3 (1984).

8 It is worth noting here that only about 3 percent of foster children go to college.

9 It is not uncommon for humans to misattribute agency, believing that they have more control over the outcome of their actions than they really do. One sociological investigation revealed that cab drivers who played craps often threw the dice harder when seeking higher numbers and with less force for lower ones, even though force in no way contributes to the probability that the roll will reveal a specific number: the chance remains one in six regardless. See James M. Henslin, "Craps and Magic," *American Journal of Sociology* 73, no. 3 (1967): 316–30. See also James M. Moore, "What Is the Sense of Agency and Why Does It Matter?" *Frontiers in Psychology* 7 (2016).

10 Here *subject* is defined as agentially antithetical to *object*. A stone, for instance, is an object because it cannot instigate action on its own, and as a result, it can change only through the actions of another. It may crack when a young boy throws it on the sidewalk, but these cracks did not come about because of any sort of agency on the part of the stone. Rather, the desire of another transformed to agency and that agency then played itself out on the stone. In contrast, the child who throws the stone remains a subject because he uses his body to express his own desire through his agency, in this case, let us say, a projected desire for destruction because his mother would not let him play with a favorite toy that represents his root desire for pleasure.

11 Alexander Quaas and Anuja Dokras, "Diagnosis and Treatment of Unexplained Infertility," *Reviews in Obstetrics and Gynecology* 1, no. 2 (Spring 2008): 69.

12 Payment varies internationally as well. See chapter 2.

13 See the National Organ Transplant Act of 1984, which bans the buying and selling of body parts: https://history.nih.gov/research/downloads/PL98-507.pdf.

14 This results in an enlargement of the ovaries from the size of walnuts to the size of oranges. Toward the end of a stimulation cycle, thin women may be able to feel or see their enlarged ovaries through the skin of their abdomen.

15 According to a 2014 report, gestational carriers accounted for 2 percent of all assisted reproductive procedures in 2005; in 2014, the number rose to 3 percent. This increase accounts only for the use of gestational surrogates in clinics in the United States and does not include the use of traditional surrogates or surrogates hired abroad by American couples, an approach discussed at greater length in chapter 2. See Centers for Disease Control and Prevention, American Society for Reproductive Medicine, Society for Assisted Reproductive

Technology, *2014 Assisted Reproductive Technology National Summary Report* (Atlanta: U.S. Department of Health and Human Services, 2016).

16 When the American Psychiatric Association first included post-traumatic stress in its diagnostic and statistical manual, it included a third criterion: that events be outside the realm of typical human experience. Rates of trauma, however, have shown that such events are unfortunately all too common. This criterion is no longer included as necessary for a diagnosis. See also Judith Herman, *Trauma and Recovery: The Aftermath of Violence—from Domestic Abuse to Political Terror* (New York: Basic Books, 1997), 33.

17 The *Diagnostic and Statistical Manual of Mental Disorders* does not delineate a set of events that qualify as traumatic but rather lists symptoms that affected individuals commonly experience. Acute or chronic post-traumatic stress disorder can be instantiated by an untold number of events, with one individual responding to a given event with different resilience than another. In other words, an event that might lead to post-traumatic stress in one individual may not lead to the same response in another. It is therefore the way an individual experiences an event that makes it traumatic, rather than an essential traumatic nature on the part of a given event itself. Still, certain events are more likely to lead to post-traumatic stress than others: an individual who departs from a friend's birthday party from which he leaves smiling and saying that the cake was the most delicious of his life and the company the most enjoyable is less likely to suffer post-traumatic stress from the birthday party than if that same individual were directly exposed to warfare. American Psychiatric Association, *Diagnostic and Statistical Manual of Mental Disorders*, 5th ed. (Washington, D.C.: American Psychiatric Publishing, 2017).

18 Infertility, for instance, if unaccompanied by another medical condition, is not life threatening. However, infertility caused by cancer is. In such cases, the cancer, and not the inability to bear children, would cause fear for one's mortality.

19 Infertility, in particular, differs in relation to other medical conditions in regards to how it manifests physically and in turn how it manifests psychologically. Many illnesses result in detrimental physical or psychological effects due either to the presence of something unwanted or the absence of something desired. Cancer requires a malignant tumor that harms the body's capability to flourish; the lack of beta cells producing insulin defines type one diabetes; too little dopamine can cause chemical depression. In these cases, the bodily malfunction results in suffering regardless of individual desire, whereas some of the suffering that occurs following a diagnosis of infertility, at least, requires the simultaneous conditions of a person desiring children and the body's inability to enact agency to reproduce.

20 Reflecting on her own miscarriage and that of a friend, Serene Jones writes that miscarriage and stillbirth create a rupture of bodily boundaries as the living body simultaneously becomes a locus of death. "We were graves. No, we weren't the dying. We would live to see another day, for sure. But that day

would be a haunted one for we also weren't simply in the world of the living, either. The site of the death we were grieving wasn't some car accident on the interstate or the cancer ward at the hospital. The space of this death wasn't a cross on a hillside where mothers wept at a distance. Nor was it some rock-hewn cave beyond the walls of Jerusalem. The death-site was inside us, deep in us. It was in a place even unknown to our eyes, in a cavern from which we had believed a future would spring forth but from which only loss had issued." Serene Jones, "Rupture," in *Hope Deferred: Heart-Healing Reflections on Reproductive Loss*, ed. Nadine Pence Frantz and Mary T. Stimming (Eugene, Ore.: Resource/Wipf & Stock, 2005), 59.

21 The experience of being a bystander in reproductive loss might be best explained as a separation from the physical part of one's self that is instantiated by the awareness that one is not in control of one's own body. In this way, the whole self fragments into a body self that is separate from the self's agency. This kind of self separation is not synonymous with the kind of dissociation that trauma survivors may experience, though dissociation may occur in reproductive trauma.

22 Quaas and Dokras, "Diagnosis and Treatment of Unexplained Infertility," 69.

23 B. J. Berg, J. F. Wilson, and P. J. Weingartner, "Psychological Sequelae of Infertility Treatment: The Role of Gender and Sex-Role Identification," *Social Science & Medicine* 33 (1991): 1071–80; P. P. Mahlstedt, "Psychological Issues of Infertility and Assisted Reproduction," *The Urologic Clinics of North America* 21 (1994): 557–66; M. Mazor, "Emotional Reactions to Infertility," in *Infertility: Medical, Emotional, and Social Considerations,* ed. M. Mazor and H. Simon (New York: Human Science Press, 1984), 23–35.

24 Maura A. Ryan notes that there can be an element of personal penalization that accompanies the quest for the meaning of infertility. She writes, "When infertility is linked to an untreated sexually transmitted disease, the effects of an abortion, the long-term use of oral contraceptives, or to a delay in childbearing on personal achievement grounds, the temptation is great to believe that one is merely now 'paying the piper,' or that God is now exacting penance for earlier sins." Maura A. Ryan, *Ethics and Economics of Assisted Reproduction: The Cost of Longing* (Washington, D.C.: Georgetown University Press, 2001), 74.

25 Such a response feeds into the beliefs of early psychoanalysts who attributed infertility and reproductive loss to unresolved psychological disorders. Psychoanalysts assumed that ambivalence about becoming a mother could contribute to reproductive difficulties. Research has largely disproved this account, instead finding that psychological disorders such as depression and anxiety increase following reproductive problems, rather than the reverse. That said, Jaffe and Diamond write that "although most clients reject the notion that their reproductive problems are because of unresolved psychological conflicts, the tendency to blame themselves for some aspect of the loss is almost universal. 'Why me?' or 'What did we do wrong?' frequently pop up in

the clinical setting. Although not always rational and almost always inaccurate, these clients find it more reassuring to blame themselves for their reproductive crisis, rather than believing it to be a random event." Janet Jaffe and Martha O. Diamond, *Reproductive Trauma: Psychotherapy with Infertility and Pregnancy Loss Clients* (Washington, D.C.: American Psychological Association, 2011), 58–59.

26 As one woman who experienced a reproductive loss reported, "I feel as if I somehow poisoned my baby, that there must have been something bad inside me. How can I ever consider getting pregnant again? This baby is gone, but the badness is still there." Jaffe and Diamond, *Reproductive Trauma*, 60.

27 Judith Herman writes that trauma tends to inaugurate an "existential crisis" in survivors as they question such assumptions—the nature of the self, systems of belief, and relationships within the community may all be called into question. Herman, *Trauma and Recovery,* 51.

28 Indeed, the stereotyped patient may have experienced financial success prior, perhaps in the professional realm, thereby giving him or her the means to undertake the procedures in the first place. That professional commitment may also have resulted in a delay in childbearing, resulting in the need for technological assistance.

29 To that end, Maura Ryan writes that the "'typical' infertility patient" is a "successful person who has achieved some measure of professional competence, who has carefully executed the various tasks of life." Ryan, *Ethics and Economics of Assisted Reproduction*, 71. For a blunter summary, Phoebe Potts describes her own reaction to an infertility diagnosis this way: "I've been steeped in the two Great American myths: You can do it. Cash is king. Combine the two and you get this easy-to-remember mantra: You can buy it! With that logic long instilled in me, I've got a classic case of middle class entitlement. . . . I married a nice (partially) Jewish boy! I recycle! I vote! I eat my greens! I go to yoga! I went to Smith! I untangled my issues in therapy! I worked for the poor! So . . . where's my baby?" Phoebe Potts, *Good Eggs* (New York: Harper, 2010), xvi–xix.

30 Essentialist reproductive anthropology may also be supported by Christian theological discourses, notably in Roman Catholic teachings on natural law.

31 Jaffe and Diamond suggest that while both men and women may be afflicted with this challenge to self-concept, women are more likely to feel that reproductive difficulties reflect some sort of inadequacy within their identity at large, perhaps because of social reinforcers within society that cause women to be more likely to feel their identity is rooted in motherhood than in other instrumental forms. Jaffe and Diamond, *Reproductive Trauma*, 60.

32 Jaffe and Diamond, *Reproductive Trauma*, 59–60.

33 Maura Ryan reflects on the process of questioning how infertility challenges the essence of gendered identity by referencing her own family's experience of infertility. She writes, "Having always thought of spiritual hospitality as a necessary virtue for the Christian theologian, especially for a feminist

theologian, it was extremely difficult, despite all I knew of the 'phenomenon,' to resist feeling that my infertility revealed not just a disorder in my reproductive system but a defect in the receptivity of my heart. Although the shape of the threat was different, our infertility also forced my husband to confront his understanding of himself as a man." Ryan, *Ethics and Economics of Assisted Reproduction*, 72.

34 Ryan, *Ethics and Economics of Assisted Reproduction*, 73. Ryan adds that infertility and reproductive loss often challenges couples to confront their personal and transgenerational mortality, and it is not uncommon for couples to feel as if they are unable to leave a lasting legacy because they cannot perpetuate the family lineage. This then makes them feel that they have not only failed at a personal level, but that they failed at a transgenerational one as well, forcing them to question their own sense of self or identity in regards to not only their premortem but also their postmortem existence. Ryan, *Ethics and Economics of Assisted Reproduction,* 72.

35 Jaffe and Diamond, *Reproductive Trauma,* 15.

36 Jaffe and Diamond, *Reproductive Trauma*, 16.

37 Psychologists Marcus and Nurius refer to this act of considering the self in the future using the term the "possible self" and suggest it is an important way of influencing how a person might develop. For instance, if a child watches *Glee* and decides she wants to sing in a high school choir, she will be more likely to ask her parents to enroll her in singing lessons and become a singer herself. In that way, the possible self becomes a reality when action is taken to enact it. Yet the concept of the possible self is also highly malleable and in flux: if child's voice teacher announces she has no sense of pitch during their first lesson together, the child may lose confidence and want to quit her lessons, instead turning to gymnastics lessons because she saw Shawn Johnson win a gold medal at the Olympics. She may then continue with gymnastics lessons until her teenage years, when the workout regime becomes too strenuous, at which point she decides to dedicate her time to gaining admission to a college far from home because she saw her brother graduate high school, move into a dorm room, and enjoy his college years. See Hazel Markus and Paula Nurius, "Possible Selves," *American Psychologist* 41 (1986): 954–69. Intriguingly, in his books *The Seasons of a Man's Life* (New York: Alfred Knopf, 1978) and *The Seasons of a Woman's Life* (New York: Alfred Knopf, 1996), psychologist Daniel J. Levinson describes a similar potential self-concept, which he terms "the Dream." The Dream, he writes, is an image of what the adult self might evolve into that develops between the ages of seventeen and twenty-three. He posits that for men, the Dream is defined by career expectations; analysis of his work on women, however, shows that the Dream is more likely to be defined by an integration of career goals and relationship goals. For an analysis of Levinson's work, see Dancy Kittrell, "A Comparison of the Evolution of Men's and Women's Dreams in Daniel Levinson's Theory of

Adult Development," *Journal of Adult Development* 5 (1998): 105–15; and Priscilla Roberts and Peter M. Newton, "Levinsonian Studies of Women's Adult Development," *Psychology and Aging* 2 (1987): 154–63.

38 See Marianne Hirsch, "Family Pictures: *Maus*, Mourning, and Post-memory," *Discourse* 15, no. 2 (1992–1993): 3–29.

39 Susan Brison coins the term "prememories" to suggest that a person may develop a vision of what appears to be an inevitable future. Though the context differs, she explains the concept in her book on rape thus: "How could one possibly remember the future? One way of trying to make sense of this paradox is to note that fear is a future-directed state and that it is primarily fear that is instilled by postmemory of rape. The backward-looking postmemory of rape thus, at every moment, turns into the forward-looking prememory of a feared future that someday *will have been*—a temporal correlate to the spatial paradox of the Möbius strip, in which what are apparently two surfaces fuse, at every moment, into one." While hopefully not fear based and, indeed, hopefully not negative in orientation at all, the concept of "prememory" indeed seems to apply to the earliest constructions of the reproductive narrative developed in childhood. Susan J. Brison, *Aftermath: Violence and the Remaking of the Self* (Princeton, N.J.: Princeton University Press, 2002), 88.

40 Though she is not writing about reproduction or in conversation with dialogues about pre- or postmemories, Carrie Doehring addresses the role of inherited narratives in the context of her work on pastoral theology. Just as prememories may result in assumptions about proper ways to inhabit reproductivity that can go unexamined because they are cultural norms, Doehring suggests that there are embedded theologies that are normative within various religious groups that may go unquestioned until individuals engage in personal discernment to address the role of these embedded theological beliefs for them. This process of discernment results in the individual deriving what Doehring terms deliberative theology, a theology that is consciously developed by the individual that may incorporate or reject previously unquestioned embedded theological beliefs. See Carrie Doehring, *The Practice of Pastoral Care: A Postmodern Approach* (Louisville: Westminster John Knox, 2015), 112–16.

41 Herman, *Trauma and Recovery*, 175–236.

42 Jaffe and Diamond, *Reproductive Trauma*, 26.

43 Burton Z. Sokoloff, "Antecedents of American Adoption," *The Future of Children* 3, no. 1 (1993): 17. Adoption remained unstructured in the United States through the eighteenth century; however, the rise of the Industrial Revolution and the influx of immigrants that accompanied it led to an increase in the number of parentless children. Whereas such children previously functioned as household servants, apprentices, or indentured servants or lived in almshouses, the public began to express a desire for a clearer understanding of these children's legal status. As a result, Massachusetts became the first state to

develop a comprehensive adoption statute, which was passed in 1851. Sokoloff, "Antecedents of American Adoption," 17–18.

44 Daniel Scott Smith, "Family Limitation, Sexual Control, and Domestic Feminism in Victorian America," in *Controlling Reproduction: An American History*, ed. Andrea Tone (Lanham, Md.: Rowman & Littlefield, 1996), 77–98.

45 The Census Bureau provides even lower numbers for single parent households. The average number of children in families raised by a mother alone is approximately 1.75, while the average number of children in families raised by a father alone is approximately 1.6. See "Figure FM-3: Average number of children per family," Families and Living Arrangements, https://www.census.gov/content/dam/Census/library/visualizations/time-series/demo/families-and-households/fm-3.pdf. It should also be noted that researchers at the Pew Research Center calculate that this number is not standard across all demographics. Maternal education, for instance, correlates to family size: mothers who have not graduated from high school, for instance, are three times more likely to have four or more children than mothers who have a postgraduate degree. Race also factors in: 20 percent of Hispanic mothers have four or more children; that number decreases to 18 percent for African American mothers, 11 percent for white mothers, and 10 percent for Asian mothers. That said, there has been a dramatic decline in fertility overall, even within each ethnic group. For example, 31 percent of Hispanic mothers had four or more children in 1988; that number had decreased to 20 percent in 2014. See Gretchen Livingston, *Childlessness Falls, Family Size Grows Among Highly Educated Women* (Washington, D.C.: Pew Research Center, 2015), http://www.pewsocialtrends.org/2015/05/07/family-size-among-mothers/.

46 It is worth noting that the U.S. government at large has a long history of separating minority children from their families, with horrific stories documented in the Native American, black, and Latino communities, among others, the most recent example of which is the separation of immigrant children at the borders of the United States. Even as these historic and contemporary examples of government-supported family separation are noted, what is being analyzed here is the *stated* mission of the Department of Children and Family Services. For a record of this statement on the current priorities of child services in regards to family reunification, see U.S. Department of Health and Human Services, "Family Reunification: What the Evidence Shows," *Child Welfare Information Gateway: Issues*, 2011, https://www.quantumunitsed.com/get-material.php?id=444.

47 The Washington State case of *Andersen v. King County* banned same-sex unions on the basis that same-sex unions cannot yield biological offspring. In the words of Washington Supreme Court Justice Barbara A. Madsen, "Limiting marriage to opposite-sex couples furthers procreation, essential to the survival of the human race, and furthers the well-being of children by encouraging families where children are reared in homes headed by the children's biological parents." Barbara A. Madsen, *Andersen v. King Decision Opinion*, July 26, 2006,

www.courts.wa.gov/newsinfo/content/pdf/759341opn.pdf, accessed October 30, 2018. See also Brian Powell, Catherine Bolzendahl, Claudia Geist, and Lala Carr Steelman, *Counted Out: Same-Sex Relations and Americans' Definitions of Family* (New York: Russell Sage Foundation, 2010), 139.

48 Powell, Bolzendahl, Geist, and Steelman, *Counted Out*, 26, 40.

49 To quote one member of the study, "A family is a married couple with children. . . . Marriage is what makes the family, it makes it legal, because you have blood to be a family if the children carry the blood." Powell, Bolzendahl, Geist, and Steelman, *Counted Out*, 41.

50 To that end, the authors of the study concluded that "the focus on blood indicates that, for exclusionists, it is not children per se who help make a family, but biological children." Powell, Bolzendahl, Geist, and Steelman, *Counted Out*, 41.

51 For an intriguing look at the intersection of feminism and natural law, see Cristina L. H. Traina, *Feminist Ethics and Natural Law: The End of the Anathemas* (Washington, D.C.: Georgetown University Press, 1999). Traina seeks to use natural law to mitigate some of the consequences of constructionism and to give a grounding to what it means to be a woman using the natural law tradition.

52 Powell, Bolzendahl, Geist, and Steelman, *Counted Out*, 41. The authors note that interviewees seemed to mention them more as an afterthought or, quoting sociologist Allen Fisher, as "still not quite as good as having your own" (49). See also Allen P. Fisher, "Still 'Not Quite as Good as Having Your Own'? Toward a Sociology of Adoption," *Annual Review of Sociology* 29 (2003): 339–51.

53 Powell, Bolzendahl, Geist, and Steelman, *Counted Out*, 41.

54 One participant summarized the views expressed by others this way, "I just feel like there's an emotional connection, emotional bonding is sometimes a tighter bond than blood." Powell, Bolzendahl, Geist, and Steelman, *Counted Out*, 56.

55 David M. Newman, *Families: A Sociological Perspective* (Boston: McGraw Hill Higher Education, 2009), 432–33.

56 Writing of her own struggles with infertility, Mary Stimming employs Tillich to suggest that the quest for biological parenthood can become a quest of ultimate concern and, in turn, function as a form of idolatry informed by American values that privilege biological parenthood to the extent that individuals assume it can provide what Tillich calls "ultimate fulfillment." Mary Stimming, "Sorrow," in Frantz and Stimming, *Hope Deferred*, 35–36.

57 Mary T. Stimming describes how the biological family may function as an idol, invoking the Tillichian definition of idol as "placing one's faith in that which is not truly ultimate." Offering theological reflection about her own inability to biologically produce a child, Stimming reflects that culture implicitly promised biological parenthood as the culmination of her reproductive future such that idolatry of the biological family did not develop in isolation but rather was embedded in "social expectations [that are] powerful amplifiers of personal desire." Stimming, "Sorrow," 36.

58 Barbara Katz Rothman, *Recreating Motherhood* (New Brunswick, N.J.: Rutgers University Press, 2000), 19.

59 It should be noted that this term is often replaced with "birth parents," precisely to delineate that parenthood is not defined by biological ties.

60 Language reinforces the ambiguity adoptive parents face because the man and woman who give up a child for adoption continue to bear the titles of birth mother and father. This grants them a lifelong parental hallmark because of their biological connection to the child. However, to say that these individuals are not parents is also reductive: while they did not take on the day-to-day task of raising the child, giving up rights to do so may well have been a difficult decision motivated by a sense of wanting what is best for the child. That sense of other-directedness, of taking steps that benefit the child even if it costs the parent, is often a characteristic of parenthood. The birth parents, especially the mother, also have the experience of a caretaking relationship with the growing infant in utero. To say that there is nothing parental about what a birth mother or father is to the child therefore seems reductive. However, that also means confusion about who is or is not a parent in cases of adoption may be natural due to multiple invocations of the terms *mother* and *father* in relationship to one particular child.

61 Rothman, *Recreating Motherhood*, 20.

62 Taken together, the fear of adopting a child with special needs and the commitment to genetics seem to indicate that parents consider children as having instrumental rather than intrinsic value. Parents' concerns about adopting children with special needs seems to signify an instrumental view of children wherein children whose bodies cannot do certain things reflects on their overall value; likewise, the child who has certain genes—namely, the genes of the intended parent—possesses value precisely because the child can be expected to have a set of qualities that emerges from those genes. In either scenario, children are not valued for being children but rather are valued for their possessed traits.

63 The data assume a twenty-four-hour/day pay scale and a thirty-one-day month.

64 See "Surrogate Mother Pay: Compensation for Surrogate Mothers," Conceive-Abilities, https://www.conceiveabilities.com/surrogates/surrogate-mother-pay, accessed March 3, 2017. See also "Surrogate Mother Compensation," Surrogacy America, https://www.surrogacyamerica.com/become-surrogate-mother/surrogate-mother-compensation, accessed March 3, 2017. Payment may increase with increased numbers of successful surrogate pregnancies. This forty-week period does not include weeks or months spent on the conception process, which would lower payment per hour.

65 White people are less likely to buy the eggs of minority donors than of white ones. The rise of medical tourism also means an increase in the number of minority surrogates. See Rothman, *Recreating Motherhood,* 26.

2 Surrogacy as Culturally Constructed

1 Sharmila Rudrappa likens Indian surrogates to garment factory workers, suggesting that surrogacy allows the Indian woman to continue to use her body productively once she can no longer work in the factory. Sharmila Rudrappa, "India's Reproductive Assembly Line," *Contexts* 11, no. 2 (2012): 22–24. Amrita Pande also strikes a comparison between the Indian surrogate and the factory worker when she notes that the Indian practice of housing surrogates in hostels and keeping them under surveillance is analogous to the housing provided to workers in former New England mill towns. Amrita Pande, *Wombs in Labor: Transnational Commercial Surrogacy in India* (New York: Columbia University Press, 2014), 81.

2 Helena Ragoné writes that the existence of surrogacy encourages a more nuanced consideration of the connection between how women's bodies function and how culture structures an understanding of their purpose. "The fact that the surrogate allows herself to be intentionally inseminated for the purpose of conceiving, bearing, and parting with a child calls for a reevaluation of biologically deterministic models, which have tended to inform cultural definitions and expectations about the perceived bond between mother and fetus and mother and child." Helena Ragoné, *Surrogate Motherhood: Conception in the Heart* (Boulder, Colo.: Westview Press, 1994), 114.

3 Ragoné, *Surrogate Motherhood*, 54.

4 Ragoné, *Surrogate Motherhood,* 54–55.

5 Ragoné, *Surrogate Motherhood,* 60–62. See also Philip Parker, "Motivations of Surrogate Mothers: Initial Findings," *American Journal of Psychiatry* 140 (1983):117–19.

6 Vivian Zelizer, *Pricing the Priceless Child* (New York: Basic Books, 1985).

7 Ragoné, *Surrogate Motherhood*, 58–59.

8 Georg Simmel, *The Philosophy of Money* (London: Routledge and Keagan Paul, 1978), 297. Ragoné troubles the discourse surrounding surrogate payment further when she writes, "Of all the surrogates' stated motivations, remuneration is the most problematic. On a symbolic level, of course, remuneration detracts from the idealized cultural image of women/mothers as selfless, nurturant, and altruistic, an image that surrogates do not wish to lose; in addition, if surrogates were to acknowledge the money as a fair and equal exchange or compensation for their reproductive work, they would lose the sense that theirs is a gift that cannot be compensated monetarily." Ragoné, *Surrogate Motherhood,* 60.

9 Ragoné, *Surrogate Motherhood,* 90–91.

10 Ragoné, *Surrogate Motherhood*, 54–55.

11 The economic disparity is particularly prominent in third-party reproductive cases that involve surrogates; egg and sperm donors tend to be assessed by not only their physical characteristics but also their intellectual, athletic, artistic, and professional achievements because of the assumption that their DNA may

be one factor in those successes. As a result, intended parents may be more likely to choose egg and sperm donors who, if they do not come from privileged backgrounds already, may ultimately come to find a place in them. In contrast, gestational surrogates are chosen not by their looks or achievements but by their bodies' ability to carry a child to term, so that a surrogate's list of achievements is far less important than evidence that she has birthed children either for herself or others before. As a result, the social and economic disparities that may exist in all third-party procedures are particularly prominent in gestational surrogacy, and the disparity between intended parents and surrogate raises the question of whether third-party procedures on the whole exploit the bodies of desperate individuals, especially desperate women.

12 Ragoné, *Surrogate Motherhood*, 22. These closed programs mirror gamete donation procedures, a majority of which remain anonymous in the United States.

13 Ragoné, *Surrogate Motherhood,* 40. See also Judith Modell, "In Search: The Purposed Biological Basis of Parenthood," *American Ethnologist* 13, no. 4 (1986): 646–61.

14 As Ragoné summarizes, "Programs reiterate (most often through individual and group therapy sessions) that the surrogate has been entrusted with an enormous amount of power and responsibility. Programs also facilitate a surrogate's desire to part with the child by emphasizing just how crucial her contribution is to a couple's future happiness. With this two-pronged approach of making the surrogate feel that if she kept the child she would destroy the lives of the couple, and fostering the idea that she has the power to make their lives joyous, a program encourages the surrogate's wish to part with the child." Ragoné, *Surrogate Motherhood*, 41.

15 As Ragoné writes, "The issue of fertility thus serves as a leveling ground for perceived, if unacknowledged, inequalities between couples and surrogates. I would suggest, tentatively, that all surrogates view their fertility to some extent as a resource that provides them with a decisive handicap or advantage in their relationship with the couple. From the surrogate's perspective, the couples' material success pales in comparison to the unhappiness their infertility and ensuing state of childlessness create in their lives. . . . Couples, because their relationship to the surrogate is firmly centered on what is lacking in their lives, rather than on their economic, educational, and social privileges, are regarded in the surrogate context as individuals who are unfulfilled and faced with a tragic impediment to the attainment of complete happiness. The issue of infertility thus serves as a pivotal and multifaceted issue in the surrogate arrangement, especially as it pertains to class differences between couple and surrogate." Ragoné, *Surrogate Motherhood*, 91–92.

16 Ragoné, *Surrogate Motherhood*, 42.

17 According to Ragoné, surrogates are not told about the couple's beliefs on such issues. Ragoné, *Surrogate Motherhood,* 42.

18 Ragoné summarizes the contrast this way, "My research shows that the couple most readily relates to their surrogate as 'the woman who is carrying our child,' and once she gives birth, they are ready to begin parenting without her assistance. The surrogate, however, relates to the couple more as friends with whom she feels a bond and from whom she has received gratitude, kindness, consideration, and respect; to the surrogate's way of thinking, that relationship should not change or end once the child has been born, no matter how well she has been prepared for this eventuality by the program." Ragoné, *Surrogate Motherhood,* 44.

19 Different perspectives concerning the termination of contact following a surrogacy procedure may imply that the surrogate perceives herself as participating in an ongoing relational contract whereas the intended parents perceive themselves as participating in a finite business contract defined by the exchange of goods.

20 Ragoné notes that clinics practicing open donation specifically instruct intended parents to be transparent with children about their origins; however, there is no way for the clinic to enforce its own requests. Ragoné cites this as just one example of ways that intended parents "flout" guidelines so that the "balance of power tilts in favor of the couples." Ragoné, *Surrogate Motherhood,* 45.

21 Stephanie O. Corley and Jessica Wilen Berg, "Embryo Donation: Ethical Issues," in *Third-Party Reproduction: A Comprehensive Guide*, ed. James M. Goldfarb (New York: Springer, 2013), 124–25. See also Lindsay Childress-Beatty, "Embryo Donation: Psychological Aspects," in Goldfarb, *Third-Party Reproduction*, 117; and Linda D. Applegarth, "Oocyte Donation: Psychological Aspects," in Goldfarb, *Third-Party Reproduction*, 43.

22 One study in the United Kingdom, for instance, found that parents rarely thought about or talked about the donors with their spouse. See Fiona MacCallum, "Embryo Donation Parents' Attitudes towards Donors: Comparison with Adoption," *Human Reproduction* 24, no. 3 (2009): 517–23.

23 Paul Lauritzen, *Pursuing Parenthood: Ethical Issues in Assisted Reproduction* (Bloomington: Indiana University Press, 1993), 84.

24 Embryo donation raises additional questions about disclosure rates, as intended parents who use donated embryos may find themselves raising children with no biological connection to them, thereby making the biological relationship with these children akin to adoption. To date, minimal studies with Americans have been conducted on disclosure rates; however, Lindsay Childress-Beatty cites British research that found that "only one-third of the embryo-donation couples had told, or were planning to tell, the child about his or her origins, in contrast to 100 percent of the adoption couples and 93 percent of the IVF couples. Almost 43 percent of the embryo-donation parents were not planning on disclosing to the child." A relatively low level of disclosure in spite of being given counseling concerning the advantages of

disclosure was also found in a Finnish sample. Childress-Beatty, "Embryo Donation," 116–17.

25 Elly Teman, *Birthing a Mother: The Surrogate Body and the Pregnant Self* (Berkeley: University of California Press, 2010), 217.

26 Amanda J. Turner and Adrian Coyle, "What Does It Mean to Be a Donor Offspring? The Identity Experiences of Adults Conceived by Donor Insemination and the Implications for Counseling and Therapy," *Human Reproduction* 15 (2000): 2041–51.

27 Writing on the legal aspects of sperm donation, Stephanie O. Corley and Maxwell Mehlman explain that "children conceived with the use of anonymous sperm are likened to adoptive children, and studies have shown that insecurities arise in adoptees because of the lack of information about the child's biological parent(s)." Stephanie O. Corley and Maxwell Mehlman, "Sperm Donation: Legal Aspects," in Goldfarb, *Third-Party Reproduction*, 154.

28 Reinforcing this data, Petok explains that children of sperm donors who discover the use of the donor later in life "can experience a disruption of identity. In essence, they are not the persons they assumed they were." As a result, he argues that "openness produces better psychological results for children conceived with donor sperm and for the families in which they are raised." William D. Petok, "Sperm Donation: Psychological Aspects," in Goldfarb, *Third-Party Reproduction*, 165–66.

29 Lauritzen, *Pursuing Parenthood*, 84–88.

30 Alexander McFarlane and Bessel van der Kolk argue that trauma survivors in general keenly feel this societal stigma and are hesitant to publicly acknowledge their experience because of the potential complications and additional suffering that can arise because of it. This occurs, they write, because "most victims who are conscious of the effects of trauma on their lives preserve their self-protective instincts and are highly ambivalent about having people find out what happened to them. For example, rape victims are usually aware that they run a great risk of not being believed, of being blamed, and of having their sexuality exposed and scrutinized. . . . Since both victims and bystanders experience intense emotions when confronted by these behaviors [traumatic responses], they are likely to lose sight of the fact that they are rooted in a past trauma. Instead, both will construct complex rationales to justify their reactions: elaborate grievances, in the case of the victims, and diagnostic constructs that invariably come to have a pejorative meaning, in the case of the bystanders. These grievances and diagnoses are designed to return a sense of control to the parties involved; ironically, however, both are likely to perpetuate the trauma in the interpersonal realm, which is dichotomized in terms of dominance and submission. After the breakdown of a healthy balance between collaboration and self-protective reserve, the resulting polarities assure that one person or group will be seen as powerful and the other as helpless. The trauma will thus continue to be played out between

helpless supplicants/victims/caregivers and predators/manipulators/oppressors. Calling victims 'survivors' is a euphemism that denies the reality of these dichotomies of powerlessness." Alexander C. McFarlane and Bessel A. van der Kolk, "Trauma and Its Challenge to Society," in *Traumatic Stress: The Effects of Overwhelming Experience on Mind, Body, and Society,* ed. Bessel A. van der Kolk, Alexander C. McFarlane, and Lars Weisaeth (New York: Guilford Press, 1996), 31–33.

31 Surrogacy is currently banned in Arizona and the District of Columbia; New York and Michigan void and penalize surrogacy. Kentucky, North Dakota, and Louisiana all declare traditional surrogacy void but allow for gestational surrogacy, while Indiana and Nebraska declare all surrogacy arrangements void. The state of Washington allows surrogacy but not monetary compensation to surrogates; Arkansas, Florida, Illinois, Nevada, New Hampshire, Texas, Utah, and Virginia all have laws allowing but regulating surrogacy arrangements. The remaining states have no laws concerning surrogacy arrangements or have bills pending as of 2017. See Magdalina Gugucheva, *Council for Responsible Genetics: Surrogacy in America* (Cambridge, Mass.: Council for Responsible Genetics, 2010), 29–40.

32 Responding to the increased use of infertility treatments coupled with the cost of them, sixteen states—Arkansas, California, Connecticut, Delaware Hawaii, Illinois, Louisiana, Maryland, Massachusetts, Montana, New York, New Jersey, Ohio, Rhode Island, Texas, and West Virginia—now have mandates that require insurers to cover infertility treatments to some extent, often covering artificial insemination or partially covering in vitro fertilization. These generally do not, however, provide for the cost of a donor or surrogate, meaning that intended parents must pay the fees and medical expenses for third parties. See https://resolve.org/what-are-my-options/insurance-coverage/infertility-coverage-state/.

33 The case resolved with the State of New Jersey recognizing the surrogate, Mary Beth Whitehead as Baby M.'s (Melissa Stern's) legal guardian, though the judge granted custody to the intended parents—Elizabeth and William Stern—on the grounds that they could provide a better home environment for Baby M. The case remains the precedent for surrogacy rulings in New Jersey.

34 In the words of one intended mother, "[In the United States] you have no idea if your surrogate mother is smoking, drinking alcohol, doing drugs. You don't know what she's doing. You have a third-party agency as a mediator between the two of you, but there's no one policing her in the sense that you don't know what's going on." Sunita Thakur, "Wombs for Rent," *Marketplace*, December 27, 2007, http://www.marketplace.org/topics/life/wombs-rent-grows-india, accessed October 30, 2018.

35 As Scott Carney writes, "Before India, only the American upper classes could afford a surrogate. . . . Now it's almost within reach of the middle class." Scott Carney, *The Red Market* (New York: William Morrow, 2011), 152.

36 Pande, *Wombs in Labor,* 20.

37 An American surrogate will get paid four to five times more than that; however, that amount does not approximate ten years' worth of work in virtually any full-time American job, even at minimum wage. By this comparative standard, therefore, one might say the Indian surrogate is better compensated. However, Carney suggests an alternative method of assessment: whereas in the United States surrogates may receive 50–75 percent of the total cost paid by parents for fertility treatments, the Indian surrogate receives only 33 percent of the total. By this rubric, the Indian surrogate is worse off than the American one. Carney, *Red Market,* 146.

38 Carney, *Red Market,* 75.

39 Scott Carney's research counters this proposal, documenting conditions in the surrogate hostels that seem to resemble the clinic more closely. He presents to readers a photograph of close to ten surrogates sharing a single bedroom, all relegated to thin mattresses, many lying in fetal positions with their hands over their heads as sun shines through a thinly curtained window. Their only source of entertainment in the homes is a single television that plays Indian soap operas. "They [surrogates] will spend their entire pregnancies under lock and key. A watchman wearing an official-looking uniform and armed with a bamboo cane monitors everyone's movements from the front gate. Visits by family members are limited but, in most cases, they are too poor to make the visit. Outdoor exercise, even a walk around the block, is a no-go. To get past the guard, the women must have an appointment at the clinic or special permission from their overseers." He concludes that the confinement program many foreigners pay for is marketed to them as a way to keep surrogates well fed; however, in reality, it is tantamount to human slavery. Carney, *Red Market,* 137.

40 Carney, *Red Market*, 76–77.

41 Pande found that all but two surrogates delivered babies for intended parents via C-section; however, all but three birthed their own children vaginally, with roughly half as many giving birth in a hospital as at home. See also Carney, *Red Market,* 140.

42 Carney, *Red Market*, 140, 147–48. Practices like these have led to conclusions like those of *New York Times* columnist Judith Warner, who writes, "What's going on in India . . . feels like a step toward the kind of insane dehumanization that filled the dystopic fantasies of Aldous Huxley's 'Brave New World' and Margaret Atwood's 'Handmaid's Tale.'" Judith Warner, "Outsourced Wombs," *New York Times*, January 3, 2008. Though no studies have been conducted, one wonders whether neonates suffer as a result of scenarios in which surrogates are poorly treated, abused, or experiencing prolonged stress due to their treatment in the confinement program. It may be, for instance, that these children may have responses similar to those documented instances of intergenerational trauma, such as those exhibited in children of Holocaust survivors who experience trauma symptoms without ever experiencing

trauma firsthand. See Tamar Bauman, "The Intergenerational Transmission of Trauma Symptoms in Children of Holocaust Survivors" (Ph.D. diss., Pace University, 2003).

43 Pande, *Wombs in Labor,* 120–21.

44 Pande, *Wombs in Labor,* 118.

45 Forced sterilization of women was common in India for nearly two decades; between 1975–1977, however, forced sterilizations of men occurred, generating enough protest to overthrow the government political party. No such protests occurred in the two decades during which women were sterilized. Pande, *Wombs in Labor,* 30–31.

46 Pande, *Wombs in Labor,* 31.

47 Ironically, the policy also means that poor, sterilized women come to clinics to inquire if there are ways for the sterilization procedures to be reversed so that they can become surrogates. Pande, *Wombs in Labor,* 31.

48 Even as the government in the contemporary United States appears to tacitly promote high birthrates for those in lower economic strata—with the consequence that it becomes more challenging for those individuals to move beyond their economic challenges—it has also historically done the reverse for vulnerable populations in the United States, with the forced sterilization of Native Americans providing a particularly strident example. What forced sterilization and policies that promote birthrates share, however, is that both negatively affect the reproductive agency of the individual; in the former case, the individual cannot choose to reproduce, whereas in the latter, the individual cannot choose not to. For more on forced sterilization of Native Americans, see Andrea Smith's *Conquest: Sexual Violence and American Genocide* (Durham: Duke University Press, 2015), 82–88.

49 India outlawed commercial surrogacy in 2017, now allowing only altruistic—unpaid—surrogacy by a consenting female family member for a heterosexual couple. See also World Health Organization (WHO) et al., *Trends in Maternal Mortality: 1990 to 2015. Estimates by the WHO, UNICEF, UNFPA, World Bank Group and the United Nations Population Division.* http://apps.who.int/iris/bitstream/10665/194254/1/9789241565141_eng.pdf. See also Pande, *Wombs in Labor,* 35.

50 Pande, *Wombs in Labor,* 118.

51 Pande, *Wombs in Labor,* 110.

52 Pande, *Wombs in Labor,* 125.

53 Teman, *Birthing a Mother,* 17.

54 Teman, *Birthing a Mother,* 18.

55 Teman, *Birthing a Mother,* 23–24.

56 This group has declined in recent years, as the government approvals committee in Israel is increasingly hesitant to allow women to participate in surrogacy if they are this impoverished. Teman, *Birthing a Mother,* 24.

57 Teman, *Birthing a Mother,* 16, 25.

58 While the Israeli health-care system covers many of surrogacy's expenses, the intended parents are still responsible for the approximately $25,000 surrogate fee, a fee of approximately $9,000 paid to the government approvals committee, $1,800 for psychological screening, and an agency fee of $8,000 if they choose to use that service. Fees therefore range between approximately $26,800 and $45,000. In contrast, costs in the United States hover at approximately $120,000 when an agency is used. Teman, *Birthing a Mother*, 24–25.
59 As in other countries, surrogates are not explicitly paid for the use of their bodies but rather are reimbursed for their time.
60 Teman, *Birthing a Mother*, 6.
61 In this regard, one might argue that the desire for the continued growth of the nation causes Jewish ethical discussions of surrogacy to exist in greater isolation from the abortion debate than it does in Christian circles.
62 Teman, *Birthing a Mother*, 12–13.
63 Teman, *Birthing a Mother*, 12.
64 A few Christian Arabs have used Israeli surrogacy, though do so in the face of strong cultural stigmas against it. No Muslims have participated, though it is worth noting that Islam forbids surrogacy. Teman, *Birthing a Mother*, 13.
65 Teman, *Birthing a Mother*, 134.
66 Teman suggests that perhaps because women who are surrogates in Israel must first be mothers of their own children, they understand the importance certain rituals can play in forming a maternal identity, and therefore they want to be sensitive to how those rituals can empower the intended mother in her maternal identity while simultaneously empowering the surrogates' role as hero.
67 As Nina, one surrogate, recounts, "I only touch it [my belly] if I feel like she [the fetus] isn't moving and I want to wake her up, to make sure that she is okay." When Teman asks Nina if she touched her belly when pregnant with her own children, she responds: "Of course. I bonded with my children. I touched them, caressed them all the time." In this example, then, one observes that Nina takes concrete actions with her body that simultaneously distance her from the mothering role while empowering the intended mother to adopt it. Teman, *Birthing a Mother*, 79.
68 One intended mother, Riki, describes how her surrogate would not allow doctors to begin procedures without her: "Even when I was thirty minutes late one time, she made him wait. She said that this is Riki's baby and that she had to be here." Teman, *Birthing a Mother*, 124.
69 Teman, *Birthing a Mother*, 82.
70 Teman, *Birthing a Mother*, 264, 266.
71 Teman, *Birthing a Mother*, 217.
72 Teman, *Birthing a Mother*, 217.
73 Teman, *Birthing a Mother*, 271. Teman here is translating from Hebrew and presumably used the shorthand G-d because the speaker honored the Jewish prohibition against saying God's name.

74 Since 2005 Israel's ministry of health has required surrogates to be admitted to gynecological wards and encouraged intended mothers' hospitalizations. However, because many hospitals want to attract business, they often absorb the cost of the intended mother's stay or ask for a small amount of money ($100 to $150 per night) for the intended mother to stay in the hospital. Teman, *Birthing a Mother*, 123–24.

75 Teman, *Birthing a Mother*, 187.

76 Teman, *Birthing a Mother*, 134.

77 Teman did not document whether it was a common Israeli practice to meet gamete donors.

3 Hagar, Sarah, and Forms of Socially Constructed Surrogacy

1 On the flip side, the woman who seeks an abortion is also negatively affected by the belief that reproduction is within human control, for it permits the argument that if she did not want to conceive, she should not have participated in intercourse in the first place, as if she consented to reproduction at the same time that she consented—assuming she did consent—to sex itself. For further discussion on the delineation between consenting to sex and consenting to reproduction, see Jarvis Thomson, "A Defense of Abortion," 47–66.

2 Delores Williams explains that it was not unusual for a slave's body to be used as a proxy for her barren mistress in matters of conception, with that proxy relationship culminating at delivery, when the slave birthed the child on the knees of her mistress, thereby transferring maternal responsibilities onto her. According to Williams, the maternal transfer was not successful in the case of Sarah. Delores S. Williams, *Sisters in the Wilderness: The Challenge of Womanist God-Talk* (Maryknoll, N.Y.: Orbis, 1993), 16. See also Gerhard von Rad, *Genesis*, trans. John H. Marks (Philadelphia: Westminster, 1956), 186.

For other examples of surrogacy in the Bible, see Gen 30:3, where Bilhah is a surrogate for Rachel, and Gen 30:9, where Zilpah is a surrogate for Leah. Ruth's child Obed is also referred to by village women as a son "born to Naomi," perhaps suggesting that Ruth served a surrogate role in that reproductive process.

3 Analysis of both Gen 16 and Gen 21 will refer to Sarah and Abraham with those names for consistency's sake, though in chapter 16, these individuals still hold their former names, Sarai and Abram. Scripture quotations are from the NRSV.

4 Kent Bach and Robert Harnish argue that the successful execution of a performative remains dependent on the receiver's execution of it, so that in this case Sarah's command to Abraham to engage in intercourse with Hagar functions as an explicit performative because of Abraham's response. Bach and Harnish thereby interpret performatives as effective contingent upon the agency of the receiver, so that in this case, Abraham's actions in response to Sarah's command determine the effectiveness—or, in Austin's terminology, felicitousness—of the performative. For more on explicit performatives, see J.

L. Austin, *How to Do Things with Words*, 2nd ed. (Oxford: Clarendon, 2011), 67–94. For more on the dependency of performatives on the receiver, see Kent Bach and Robert M. Harnish, *Linguistic Communication and Speech Acts* (Cambridge, Mass.: MIT Press, 1979).

5 Johanna H. Stuckey notes that it is important to remember that female goddesses such as Inanna-Ishtar (Meospotamian), Anat (Canaanite), Asherah (Canaanite and Israelite), or Hera (Greek) did not exist in goddess-oriented cultures but rather in patriarchal ones that included female deities due to their polytheistic worship structure. Within these cultures, female deities were likely worshipped in folk—and not state—religious rituals. There is not anything like uniformity among the goddesses in relation to their identities or responsibilities; many were responsible for fertility, though not all were wives or mothers. Stuckey also hypothesizes that the identity of goddesses became more maternal over time, as in the case of Inanna and Hera. Stuckey also provides analysis of the reinterpretation of female goddess power using images of Stone Age figurines—perhaps goddesses themselves—who appear without children, whereas children began appearing during the New Stone Age or Neolithic Age as farming came to prominence. Stuckey's interpretation of the figurines is that the solidification of patriarchy arose alongside the prominence of women as mother goddesses during this period. See Johanna H. Stuckey, "Ancient Mother Goddesses and Fertility Cults," *Journal of the Association for Research on Mothering* 7, no. 1 (2005): 32–44.

6 Candida Moss and Joel Baden argue that while fertility was a blessing in the ancient world, it was God who opened and closed the womb, such that the inability to have children was not a punishment so much as the natural state of a woman. Moss and Baden, *Reconceiving Infertility*, 55–58.

7 This argument holds only if Hagar is a slave woman and not handmaid or wife. See the following section on Hagar's identity.

8 Williams, *Sisters in the Wilderness*, 4.

9 Nelson Mandela, *Long Walk to Freedom: The Autobiography of Nelson Mandela* (Boston: Little, Brown, 1994), 624.

10 The child of a slave in ancient Israelite culture could potentially have inherited from the slaveholder, provided that the slaveholder laid parental claim to the child. See the following section on Hagar's identity.

11 Wilda Gafney suggests, to this end, that Sarah finds herself in a liminal place of simultaneously holding a degree of power even as she also exists in a position of subservience. "Sarah's actions evoke both complicity with dominant male abuse of subordinated women and the independent abusive actions of dominant-culture women against subordinated women. The legacies of the relationship tropes among Hagar, Sarah, and Abraham survive them and transcend their cultures of origin." Wilda Gafney, *Womanist Midrash: A Reintroduction to the Women of the Torah and the Throne* (Louisville: Westminster John Knox, 2017), 44.

12 Jo Ann Hackett argues that it is difficult if not impossible to write a history of women because there is a "timeless" quality to women's identity as mothers and wives, so that there is, in effect, no history to write because of their static state of being. See Jo Ann Hackett, "Can a Sexist Model Liberate Us? Ancient Near Eastern 'Fertility' Goddesses," *Journal of Feminist Studies in Religion* 5, no. 1 (1989): 65–66.

13 Williams, *Sisters in the Wilderness*, 82–83; Elizabeth Bettenhausen. "Hagar Revisited: Surrogacy, Alienation, and Motherhood," *Christianity and Crisis* 47 (May 1987): 157–59.

14 In addition to arguing that Hagar's name is more properly conceived as an epithet and not a proper name, Wilda Gafney also notes that the Islamic tradition names Hagar slightly differently—Hajar—and that this shift results in an entirely different meaning of her name. "The range of potential meanings for Hajar's name includes 'splendid' and 'nourishing' in the wider cognate Semitic language system." Gafney, *Womanist Midrash,* 40–41.

15 See Philip Y. Yoo, "Hagar the Egyptian: Wife, Handmaid, and Conclubine," *Catholic Biblical Quarterly* 78 (2016): 223.

16 Scholars debate the relationship between the Hebrew terms for *handmaid* (אמה) and *slave* (שפחה), as some evidence suggests the terms are synonymous while others suggest a distinction. Within the Hebrew Bible, the appearance of these terms in 1 Sam 25:41; 2 Sam 14:15, and the Holiness Code in Leviticus (19:10; 25:6, 44) presents the terms as synonymous. Other scholars such as Chaim Cohen suggest a difference in derivation but not meaning between the terms, while Ingrid Riesener suggests the difference has to do with the type of work a woman performs. Yoo concludes, specifically in relation to an analysis of the Hagar story, that the term אמה does signify greater privilege and legal protection than שפחה. See Baruch J. Schwartz, "A Literary Study of the Slave-Girl Pericope—Leviticus 19:20-22," *Studies in the Bible, Scripta Hierosolymitana* 31, ed. Sara Japhet (Jerusalem: Magnes, 1986): 241–55. See also Baruch J. Schwartz, *The Holiness Legislation: Studies in the Priestly Code* (Jerusalem: Magnes, 1999), 330; Chaim Cohen, "Studies in Extra-biblical Inscriptions I: The Semantic Range and Usage of the Terms אמה and שפחה," *Shnaton* 5–6 (1982–1983): xxi–liii; and Ingrid Riesener, *Der Stamm* עָבַר *im Alten Testament: Eine Wortuntersuchunt unter Berucksichtigun neuerer sprachwissenschaftlicher Methoden*, Beihefte zur Zeitschrift für die Alttestamentliche Wissenschaft 149 (Berlin: de Gruyter, 1979), 76–83. See also Yoo, "Hagar the Egyptian," 227–31.

17 Hammurabi's Code states that if a first wife and slave woman both bear children from the first wife's husband, and if the husband treats both children as his own, then inheritance would be divided between the slave and first wife upon the husband's death; if the father does not refer to both sets of children as his own, then only the child of the first wife will receive an inheritance. See Yoo, "Hagar the Egyptian," 225–26. Kayla White also notes that a second wife could be constructed in two different ways in ancient times, as reflected

in ancient marriage contracts. A husband would sometimes marry sisters in order to mitigate the possibility of barrenness. The legal contracts derived from such marriages often allowed the children of one wife to be considered the children of the other; in the case of the divorce of one, the other would be divorced as well, so that the wives received mutual protection, as the loss of two dowries would likely be financially devastating for the husband. In contrast, a husband could "adopt" a second wife, but this woman would remain a slave to the first wife. In such cases, the first wife still has authority over the second wife and can send her away from the home. This scenario seems to align more with what is described in the relationship between Sarah and Hagar. See Kayla White, "The Legal Status of Barren Wives in the Ancient Near East," *Priscilla Papers* 28, no. 4 (2014): 19.

18 Philip Y. Yoo concludes that Hagar's conflicting identities can only be reconciled through source-critical analysis of Gen 16 and Gen 21, which reveals that the three terms used to describe Hagar are best attributed to three different sources, each corresponding to exclusive use of one of the three terms. J composed Gen 16:1-2, 4-14 and refers to Hagar as slave (שפחה); P composed Gen 16:3-4, which refers to Hagar as wife (אשה); and E composed Gen 21:9-21, which refers to Hagar as a handmaid (אמה). The redactor combined these stories without altering the adjectives used to describe Hagar, creating a nuanced, if confusing, picture of her identity. See Yoo, "Hagar the Egyptian," 231, 235.

19 I am indebted to conversations with Jane Patterson, in which she provided valuable insights about the possibilities that the nuance and significance of these biblical Hebrew terms have for modern-day surrogacy.

20 For extensive discussion of Hagar's voice, see the chapter "Hagar: The Desolation of Rejection" in Phyllis Trible, *Texts of Terror: Literary-Feminist Readings of Biblical Narratives* (Philadelphia: Fortress, 1984), 9–36.

21 Trible suggests ambiguity in the Hebrew verb קלל, which is used to describe the way that Hagar looked at Sarah after discovering the pregnancy. As Trible writes, "The Hebrew expression, 'her mistress was slight (or trifling) in her eyes' inspires various interpretations. Many translators alter the syntax to make Hagar the subject of the verb. They also attribute the verb (*qll*) the legitimate, though not necessary meaning of contempt or disdain." As a result, some translations suggest that Hagar looked at Sarah with "contempt" following her impregnation, while others translate the verb to give it a less bitter connotation. See Trible, *Texts of Terror,* 12.

22 Trible, *Texts of Terror*, 16.

23 Wilda Gafney reads this text with a stronger condemnation of divine direction, proposing that God's order to Hagar to return to Sarah and Ishmael after her first wilderness departure symbolizes how religious communities may be apt to privilege abusers at the expense of the abused. Such an interpretation allows for a relevant contemporary reading of the text, though it may challenge a reader who affirms God as all good. See Gafney, *Womanist Midrash*, 44.

24 As Delores Williams reads the text, Sarah's feelings toward Hagar intimate something about Sarah's maternal relationship with Ishmael: "If Ishmael could claim his right of primogeniture, Hagar's power and status could only increase. Most of what is presented in the text suggests that Ishmael was the son of Abraham and Hagar was regarded as mother, since Sarah appears not to have taken him. . . . This concern of Sarah's about inheritance seems to reinforce the idea that she has not accepted Ishmael and thus could not expect the care from him that adopted children were supposed to render their parents in their old age." Williams, *Sisters in the Wilderness,* 28.

25 The Muslim interpretation of this story differs geographically from the Judeo-Christian one. Paran is often thought to be part of the Sinai Peninsula for the Jewish and Christian communities, though the exact site is unknown. The Muslim tradition locates Paran near Mecca. In the Muslim tradition, Hajar searches for a well in the wilderness of Paran and finds one at Zamzam; to commemorate the way that God satisfied Hajar and Ishmael's thirst, pilgrims visit the well at Zamzam as part of the hajj.

26 Trible observes that only in this second wilderness departure does Hagar linguistically seem to hold subjectivity. "Of the few fragments [in Genesis] that disclose Hagar's story, this section alone (21:14e-16) depicts her apart from all other major characters. Though the child is dying, the narrated focus remains steadily on the mother: her actions, her thoughts, her words, her emotions. With one minor exception (21:15a), she is the subject of every verb." Trible writes, "But her powerless is present in the absence of her name. Moreover, as subject she is also object, having been cast out into the wilderness." Trible, *Texts of Terror,* 25.

27 Williams takes much of this analysis from the scholarship of Roland de Vaux, who writes, "To be without family is to be without protection." Roland de Vaux, *Ancient Israel: Its Life and Institutions*, trans. John McHugh (London: Darton, Longman & Todd, 1961), 85. Williams, *Sisters in the Wilderness,* 30.

28 Lee Anna Starr, *The Bible Status of Women* (New York: Fleming H. Revell, 1926), 67. See also Williams, *Sisters in the Wilderness,* 33. Williams postulates that the offspring from Ishmael and his Egyptian wife resulted in the founding of a new house, named not after a man—as was traditionally done—but after Hagar herself. Hence, just as Midian founded the Midianites and Reuben the Reubenites, so Hagar founded a tribe called the Hagarites, creating a lasting legacy for herself in the form of a house.

29 See Trible, *Texts of Terror,* 25.

30 Moss and Baden, *Reconceiving Infertility,* 40. Wilda Gafney likewise reflects that earlier in the narrative, Hagar has one source of power—her fertility—but as a slave, she has no power over how that fertility gets used. Gafney, *Womanist Midrash,* 41.

31 Williams fashions the story of Hagar as a prototype for the experiences of historical and contemporary African American women, summarizing that

Hagar's journey symbolizes "the faith, hope and struggle with which an African slave woman worked through issues of survival, surrogacy, motherhood, rape, homelessness and economic and sexual oppression." Williams, *Sisters in the Wilderness,* 33.

32 JoAnne Marie Terrell's struggle with the cross, salvation, and victimization is useful here. In contrast with the assertion Delores Williams makes that there is nothing salvific in suffering—on the cross, in black women's experience, or otherwise—Terrell states that God's decision to be "*at-one*" with humans through the cross is of positive value, especially for those in the midst of suffering: "I believe that the continuous intercession of the spirit of Christ must become integral to womanist reckonings of Christ Jesus' significance. Not the resurrection but Christ's intercession signals the end of the gospel story and the beginning of Christ's significance for us." JoAnne Marie Terrell, *Power in the Blood? The Cross in the African American Experience* (Eugene, Ore.: Wipf & Stock, 2005), 125.

33 Williams offers a more optimistic reading in which Hagar's story symbolizes that a person in a state of powerlessness who lacks supportive human relationships can achieve a unique degree of greatness. As the founder of a new house, Hagar ultimately becomes a woman who reclaims her identity as subject instead of object, a subject who emerges from a place where she could not express desire or exert agency to a place where she can. Having said that, Williams is not offering a theology of redemptive suffering. Williams wants to drive home the theological point that while God can offer a redemptive future after an experience of surrogacy, this in no way redeems surrogacy itself. There is no positive value to surrogacy for Williams, and any redemption that God offers in no way directly redeems the negative value of surrogacy itself. By proxy, there is nothing redemptive in the suffering Jesus experiences on the cross, though the resurrection God facilitates in its aftermath has redemptive value. Finally, the suffering black women experience in literal or metaphoric surrogacy, coerced or voluntary, is not redemptive. No good comes from their harm; whatever redemption God offers is extrinsic to the harm itself, for to say otherwise would be a justification of the injustices society inflicts on black women.

This reading contrasts substantially with the one offered by Trible, which suggests that the second expulsion into the wilderness is ultimately more harmful to Hagar than the first because of the role that God's rejection plays in the narrative, especially when compared with the way that God engaged with the ancient Israelites during their own expulsion into the wilderness by the Egyptian Pharaoh. From Trible's perspective, Hagar's expulsion parallels that of the ancient Israelites, with both being thrown into the wilderness. However, Hagar is an Egyptian woman who is expelled by Israelites, whereas the Israelites were collectively expelled by the Egyptian ruler. God ultimately provides ongoing support for the Israelites but does not extend the same support to Hagar and Ishmael. See Williams, *Sisters in the Wilderness,* 15–37; and Trible, *Texts of Terror,* 23–29.

34 Williams explicitly takes issue with this construct for surrogacy, especially with its self-sacrificial overtones, arguing that sacrifice does not procure salvation, either for the black woman or for Jesus, who she argues functions as a surrogate. She makes the argument thus, "Jesus represents the ultimate surrogate figure; he stands in the place of someone else: sinful humankind. Surrogacy, attached to this divine personage, thus takes on an aura of the sacred. It is therefore fitting and proper for black women to ask whether the image of a surrogate-God has salvific power for black women or whether this image supports and reinforces the exploitation that has accompanied their experience with surrogacy. . . . Can there be salvific power for black women in Christian images of oppression (for example, Jesus on the cross) meant to teach something about redemption?" Williams, *Sisters in the Wilderness*, 161–62. For contrasting womanist views of sacrifice, see Baker-Fletcher's analysis of Mamie Till-Mobley in *Dancing with God: The Trinity from a Womanist Perspective* (St. Louis: Chalice, 2006), 142; and Traci C. West's vision of the menstruating Christ in "When a White Man-God Is the Truth and the Way," in *Christology and Whiteness: What Would Jesus Do?* ed. George Yancy (New York: Routledge, 2012), 124.

35 Studies find that a majority of surrogates hold altruistic motives—namely, they state that they want to help a childless couple. For a minority, finances are the primary motivation. This finding holds across contexts where surrogates are paid—as in the United States—and in contexts where they are not, such as the United Kingdom. See Eric Blyth, "'I Wanted to Be Interesting. I Wanted to Be Able to Say "I've Done Something Interesting with My Life"': Interviews with Surrogate Mothers in Britain," *Journal of Reproductive and Infant Psychology* 12 (1994): 189–98; V. Jadva, C. Murray, E. Lycett, F. MacCallum, and S. Golombok, "Surrogacy: The Experiences of Surrogate Mothers," *Human Reproduction* 18 (2003): 2196–204; and Melinda M. Hohman and Christine B. Hagan, "Satisfaction with Surrogate Mothering," *Journal of Human Behavior in the Social Environment* 4 (2001): 61–84.

36 For more-expansive explorations of being an ally in various contexts, see the definitions of the term provided by Shannon Craigo-Snell, Christopher Doucot, and Marilyn McCord Adams in Shannon Craigo-Snell and Christopher Doucot, *No Innocent Bystander: Becoming an Ally in the Struggle for Justice* (Louisville: Westminster John Knox), 3, 84–85.

37 For more on how the virtues generally relate to being an ally, see Craigo-Snell and Doucot, *No Innocent Bystander,* 71–93.

38 Pande, *Wombs in Labor,* 124–25.

39 Pande, *Wombs in Labor,* 104–11.

40 Pande, *Wombs in Labor,* 111.

41 Sharon Jacob observes that while Indian surrogates appear to engage in acts of resistance, this resistance has the dubious honor of "being experienced only in their consent to exploitation exemplified through the capitalization of their reproductive services." While this seems unideal, one is left asking whether a

scenario for resistance exists in which the party exercising resistance is not, in some way, disadvantaged. Here again the image of ally may make more sense to employ, for an ally participates in resistance not because of the personal experience of being disadvantaged in a certain way but out of solidarity for the class that is. Sharon Jacob, *Reading Mary alongside Indian Surrogate Mothers: Violent Love, Oppressive Liberation, and Infancy Narratives* (New York: Palgrave Macmillan, 2015), 96–97.

42 Pande summarizes the irony well when she writes, "The embodied labor performed by the surrogates subverts anti-natalist state propaganda and hegemonic narratives that frame the reproductive bodies of poor women as wasteful. At the risk of undermining the power of these subversive narratives, however, I urge readers to notice the unintended consequences of these resistances at the discursive and individual levels. In essence, individual resistances have unintended consequences whereby challenges to one form of domination almost inevitably lead to reification of another. Thus while the embodied labor that the surrogates undertake is an indication of creative resistance and of the ability of a group of women to convert their 'wasteful' motherhood (as historically portrayed by the state) to productive motherhood (in terms of their ability to use their bodies to earn income), it is inherently paradoxical in nature. As these women align their own reproduction, through decisions about fertility, sterilization, and abortion, in order to (re)produce children of higher classes and privileged nations, they are fulfilling the global imperative of reducing the fertility of lower-class women in the global south." Pande, *Wombs in Labor,* 23.

43 Catherine Keller, "Delores Williams: Survival, Surrogacy, Sisterhood, Spirit," *Union Seminary Quarterly* 58, nos. 3–4 (Fall 2004): 86–88.

44 Hagar's first casting into the wilderness becomes, in Catherine Keller's reading of Williams, the first step in liberation precisely because God offers in that moment an opportunity for Hagar to recognize that her very survival signifies the possibility that something more significant exists for her, even as she simultaneously recognizes God upholding the covenant with Abraham. That first casting out therefore represents multivalence within Hagar's surrogacy experience—her surrogacy is simultaneously an abuse even as it affords her an opportunity for a freedom she might not have had without it. There is, then, a positive element to resistive surrogacy, even as that positive element may be far from archetypal.

According to Keller, "Williams' theology of survival may seem like quite a come-down from the jubilant mood of liberation. Survival might seem to come with a 'mere' front. . . . Worse, God in Gen 16 and Gen 21 'sides with Sarah,' Hagar's oppressor, and affirms the covenant with Abraham at Hagar's expense. This is a tough-minded reading (and certainly tough for many of my students, among them African American women). . . . God opens our eyes that we may *see*—and then *do* what we can and need to do. . . . Surrogacy is *both* the site of Hagar's oppression *and* of her survival, her vision, and her ultimate wellbeing. This shifty signifier of surrogacy indeed resembles the 'productive ambivalence' of postcolonial theory: possibility opens within oppression." Keller, "Delores Williams: Survival, Surrogacy, Sisterhood, Spirit," 86–88 (emphasis in original).

45 The cases of surrogacy that Williams describes in the historical and contemporary lives of African American women may best be situated under the heading of injurious surrogacy, causing harm that exists in isolation from the possibility of a salvific response. See Williams, *Sisters in the Wilderness,* 32–75.

46 The shift from injurious to constructive surrogacy does not occur for the African American woman in Williams' reading, nor does it occur for Jesus as a metaphoric surrogate. In both of those cases, the power dynamics of the overarching system in which the surrogates operate remains static, such that there is no possibility that participants could engage with surrogacy in a resistive or constructive way. This leads Williams to argue against redemptive value in the cross, situating it instead exclusively in the resurrection. Williams, *Sisters in the Wilderness,* 143–58.

4 The Self, Corporate Sin, and Cultural Misorientation

1 Studies find that surrogates report increased dissatisfaction with the outcome of surrogacy if contact with the intended parents decreases. Reame, Kalfoglou, and Hanafin found that 60 percent of surrogates did not have contact with parents or the child following surrogacy and reported disappointment; they also stated that parents desired the termination of contact but that they did not. A more recent longitudinal study by Jadva, Blake, and Casey found that 60 percent of surrogates maintained contact with families after the pregnancy, with 75 percent reporting satisfaction with the level of interaction they had. See N. E. Reame, A. Kalfoglou, and H. A. Hanafin, "Long Term Outcomes of Surrogate Pregnancy: A Report of Surrogate Mother's Satisfaction, Life Events and Moral Judgements Ten Years Later," *Fertility and Sterility* 70 (1988): 28–29; and V. Jadva et al, "Surrogacy Families 10 Years On: Relationship with the Surrogate, Decisions over Disclosure and Children's Understanding of Their Surrogacy Origins," *Human Reproduction* 27 (2012): 3008–14.

2 For an anecdotal example of the power of doctors to manipulate hope in the reproductive process, see Peggy Orenstein, *Waiting for Daisy: A Tale of Two Continents, Three Religions, Five Infertility Doctors, an Oscar, an Atomic Bomb, a Romantic Night, and One Woman's Quest to Become a Mother* (New York: Bloomsbury, 2008), 177–78.

3 This definition of sin as systemic and culturally inherited—rather than individual and sexually transmitted—aligns with that of many other contemporary theologians, especially those whose work locates itself within feminist or liberation theology conversations. For an overview of prominent work in social sin from these perspectives, see Derek R. Nelson, *What's Wrong with*

Sin: Sin in Individual and Social Perspective from Schleiermacher to Theologies of Liberation (New York: T&T Clark, 2009), 83–159.

4 Letty Russell provides a useful analysis of the Sarah and Hagar story that acknowledges the influence of systemic oppression on Hagar. It does not, however, discuss the role that systemic oppression might have played—albeit in a significantly different way—in Sarah's life and consequent decision-making process. See Letty M. Russell, *Church in the Round: Feminist Interpretation of the Church* (Louisville: Westminster John Knox, 1993), 27–29.

5 For a consideration of how social, corporate, or systemic sin can be construed in the classical language of "missing the mark," see Craigo-Snell and Doucot, *No Innocent Bystander,* 59–61.

6 See Stimming, "Sorrow," 36, for a more extensive discussion of the biological family as theological idol. In addition, for a theological and historical examination of contextual influence on the family, especially the influence of the context of Christianity, see Rosemary Radford Ruether, *Christianity and the Making of the Modern Family* (Boston: Beacon Press, 2000).

7 For a policy analysis of assisted reproduction and adoption, specifically focusing on ways that policies promote the former while not supporting the latter, see Elizabeth Bartholet, *Family Bonds: Adoption, Infertility, and the New World of Child Reproduction* (Boston: Beacon Press, 1999).

8 Nadine Pence Frantz note how mourning becomes central to acknowledging the loss of hope that results in self-objectification. See "Why?" in Frantz and Stimming, *Hope Deferred,* 25–27.

9 Mary T. Stimming offers personal reflection and theological analysis of how infertility and reproductive loss can challenge the knowledge of one's identity as a child of God; she notes that assumptions about her identity and the hopes she had for that identity had to transmogrify in the wake of reproductive difficulties, causing her to recognize how the biological family construct influenced her own perception of herself and the perception others had of her. She also acknowledges that the Church may have a uniquely prophetic voice in this regard, offering a reminder that the self is grounded in *imago Dei* even as the secular world challenges that belief.

Stimming's analysis inevitably leads to the question of what significance an event like reproductive loss or infertility has on the self if it does not define the self. Speaking about theological anthropology from a different context—specifically the context of war and cultural violence—Miroslav Volf argues that any trauma the self experiences is forgotten in the afterlife precisely because the self is not defined by worldly events but by humans' participation in the *imago Dei*. However, one is left asking what the purpose of any negative event is for the self if it does not bear lasting or even significant impact on the individual. In other words, what is gained by a negative event that is worth its cost to the individual, if it does not form or affect the individual in any theologically significant way?

One way to resolve this issue would be to recognize that to be *imago Dei* encompasses being *imago Christi* such that the suffering experienced by Christ becomes part of the suffering experienced by God. Such a theology holds sway only insofar as suffering, particularly the suffering on the cross, is part of the salvific event that culminates in the resurrection. Within such a theological framework, suffering receives its meaning because it helps form the self in a way that finds its ultimate meaning and purpose in either literal or metaphoric resurrection. However, this analysis leads to a host of theodicy-based questions and inconsistencies that extend beyond the topic at hand.

See Stimming, "Sorrow," in Frantz and Stimming, *Hope Deferred*, 33–45, and Miroslav Volf, *The End of Memory: Remembering Rightly in a Violent World* (Grand Rapids: Eerdmans, 2006).

10 The dignity of the human being also grounds Roman Catholic theological discussion of assisted reproduction, though restored agency does not. Roman Catholic documents therefore take analysis of human dignity of the person who is unable to reproduce in a different direction, advocating for adoption and childless living instead of allowing for any form of assisted reproduction. This moral guidance largely stems from the Roman Catholic Church's belief that human dignity originates at conception and extends until natural death, such that assisted reproduction of any sort becomes forbidden because of the creation of embryos during the process and their potential treatment that the Church regards as contrary to the embryo's dignity, including the freezing of the embryo or the willful discarding of embryos. For more on the Roman Catholic Church's perspective on assisted reproductions, see the Vatican instructions *Donum vitae* and *Dignitas personae.* Congregation for the Doctrine of the Faith, *Donum vitae;* Congregation for the Doctrine of the Faith, *Dignitas personae.*

11 For more on how reproductive loss and infertility violate agency, see Frantz, "Why?" in Franz and Stimming, *Hope Deferred*, 25.

12 For a deeper analysis of teaching as motherhood, see Monica Coleman's essay, which proposes that teaching is a form of "working motherhood." "Sacrifice, Surrogacy, and Salvation: Womanist Reflections on Motherhood and Work," *Black Theology* 12, no. 3 (2014): 200–212.

13 However, even in such circumstances, exploitation is usually not what intended parents primarily seek but rather is a by-product of their desire to have a family. This becomes part of the tragedy of cultural misorientation, that in seeking to reassert themselves as subjects or to exert agency, intended parents thwart the subjectivity or agency in another so that the cycle of objectivity and subverted agency perpetuates.

14 In this way, the intended parent in contemporary reproduction differs somewhat from the slaveholder Williams describes. Whereas the slaveholder is primarily motivated by economics and is willing to turn the slave into an object as a result, the intended parent's motivation is primarily a desire to make good

on their experience of alienation in a way that the slaveholder is not. In this way, the slaveholder seeks to alienate the slave; the intended parent is trying to navigate his or her own experience of alienation, and, in so doing, has the potential to alienate others as a result.

15 Marilyn McCord Adams, *Horrendous Evils and the Goodness of God* (Ithaca, N.Y.: Cornell University Press, 1999).

16 Marilyn McCord Adams, "Friendliness, Divine and Human" in *Rethinking the Medieval Legacy for Contemporary Theology*, ed. Anselm K. Min (Notre Dame, Ind.: University of Notre Dame: 2014), 43–71.

17 Adams here contrasts with Volf's view of meaning-making. According to Volf, humans will forget their premortem experiences in the afterlife because those experiences do not ultimately shape their identity in relation to the divine, nor can the power of those experiences overshadow a postmortem experience of the divine. At stake in the distinction is the role of premortem life for the individual's identity, with Adams arguing that premortem experiences of suffering, ecstasy or anything in between essentially shape the individual's identity in a way that Volf does not allow. This, in turn, leads to the question of the purpose of premortem suffering or premortem joy: if, as Volf suggests, the individual is defined purely in relationship to God, then one can ask what is gained by premortem experiences that serves any kind of substantive purpose. In relation to suffering in particular, one may ask what is gained by suffering that makes suffering worth the cost. See Volf, *The End of Memory*, 152–215.

18 Here Adams is not saying that material creation is inherently faulty but rather that within the goodness of creation are vulnerabilities that crack open the possibility for horrendous evils to break through. These vulnerabilities can, in turn, affect the divine–human relationship: "I begin with the assumption that in the world as we know it the human condition is nonoptimal and divine–human relations are nonoptimal. My own diagnosis of the root of our nonoptimality problems is that God has made us material persons in a material world of real and apparent scarcity, and that this situation makes us radically vulnerable to horrendous evils." *Horrendous Evils*, 53.

19 For a short biblical analysis of the significance of thinking about God as friend, see Elisabeth Moltmann-Wendell, "Motherhood or Friendship," in *The Power of Naming: A Concilium Reader in Feminist Liberation Theology*, ed. Elisabeth Schüssler Fiorenza (London: SCM Press, 1996).

20 The different significance of desire and agency in surrogacy may be one reason feminists hold divided perspectives on it, with some seeing it as a way for women to achieve their own liberation and to more fully live into their sense of vocation or embodied essence while others view it as inherently suppressive. Similar dichotomies of opinion exist in feminist discussions of prostitution and headscarves, both of which involve a complex interplay between individual bodies, individual desires, individual agency, and overarching cultural constructs. Pande includes analysis of surrogacy as it parallels feminist conversations

about prostitution in *Wombs in Labor.* For an extensive analysis of feminist perspectives of headscarves, see Saba Mahmood, *Politics of Piety: The Islamic Revival and the Feminist Subject* (Princeton, N.J.: Princeton University Press, 2012).

21 Franco, Blau, and Zimbardo categorize three types of heroes: military heroes who undertake physical risks, bound by duty; civilian heroes who take physical risks without being bound by duty; and social heroes, who do not necessarily undertake short-term physical risk but nonetheless experience some form of risk and sacrifice "in other dimensions of life, including serious financial consequences, loss of social status, possible long-term health problems, and social ostracism." Zeno E. Franco, Kathy Blau, and Philip G. Zimbardo, "Heroism: A Conceptual Analysis and Differentiation between Heroic Action and Altruism," *Review of General Psychology* 15, no. 2 (2011): 99–113.

22 Franco, Blau, and Zimbardo, "Heroism," 6, 26.

23 Franco, Blau, and Zimbardo, "Heroism," 6, 8. Franco, Blau, and Zimbardo categorize ten subtypes of social heroes, two of which may apply to the surrogate: the Good Samaritan and the Odds Beater/Underdog. The authors suggest Good Samaritans help others in need despite disincentives for altruistic behavior, while the Odds Beater/Underdog overcomes difficulties to provide a model for others. Both subtypes resonate with how surrogates have defined their own actions.

24 By way of hypothetical example, imagine a person who is told that her brother will be run over by a train unless she pulls a lever. Also, if she pulls the lever, she will receive a penny. The person loves her brother and pulls the lever because she loves him so much that she does not want him to die. She takes the penny not because the penny motivated her to pull the lever but because it was part of the deal. This is, of course, a far different example from the type of commitment and remuneration described in surrogacy, but it offers an explanation of how it is possible to be motivated by altruism and receive payment. Helping professions, however, might be more realistic parallels: a teacher or a nurse might genuinely choose such a profession because he enjoys nurturing children or healing the sick. The money may be important to this individual, but given that the individual could have been paid to do a number of things, it is not the money that motivates the individual but the altruistic elements of the job itself.

25 One might also counter that this vision of the social hero is a distinctly Western one and that notions of heroism may look quite different across cultures. Franco, Blau, and Zimbardo suggest this is an area for further research, acknowledging that their study—while it engaged participants from five continents—was still composed primarily of Western participants, a majority of whom were white. Franco, Blau, and Zimbardo, "Heroism," 15.

26 This framework of social hero starkly contrasts with the conditions Williams describes in her evaluation of surrogacy, conditions in which desires cannot not be freely enacted and choices cannot be freely made. In such conditions,

it is right to conclude that surrogacy functions in an exploitive manner that harms the self of the surrogate. What separates Williams' description of African American surrogates from the surrogate as social hero is not only the role of agency but also the societal view of the surrogate: the African American woman coerced into surrogacy was also coerced into a societal position that kept her subservient and powerless. Those with power, therefore, used surrogacy to control the African American woman. In contrast, the social hero not only freely acts but receives validation for her choice.

27 While one motivation for outlawing anonymous surrogacy is that it prevents children from gaining important genetic information, another might be that relationships between third parties and intended parents who choose to practice anonymously do not develop during the course of the procedures. Elly Teman comments that encouraging intended parents and third parties to develop relationships helps all participants to feel validated during the procedures and prevents commodification of the reproductive process. However, American clinics currently do not seem to prioritize such relationship cultivation in the same way Israeli clinics do. As Teman explains specifically in relation to surrogacy, "Many U.S. commercial agencies explicitly formulate the contractual *agreement* in terms of a business contract and 'educate' their surrogates to view surrogacy as a paid job." Teman, *Birthing a Mother,* 198.

28 Williams analyzes at length the metaphoric dimension of surrogacy in her discussion of the historic and contemporary experiences of African American women and uses that analysis to conclude that surrogacy is de facto damaging because those with power force those without power to carry burdens—be it the physical weight of a developing child or the metaphorical weight of increased labor—that ought to be undertaken by themselves. Yet perhaps she is saying less about surrogacy qua surrogacy than she is saying about societies that collectively construct themselves in such a way that the amount of power one has is intended to reflect the amount of value one has. It points to the danger that emerges when the collective constructs dignity instrumentally as opposed to intrinsically, and as a result, harmful instantiations of surrogacy perhaps reflect more about the community than they do about the value surrogacy can potentially have for one woman who bears a child for another. However, until an example emerges of a society that fully allows surrogates to agree to participate in reproduction freely, motivated by their own sense of vocation or charism and with the broader community acknowledging the surrogate's worth and intrinsic value, it will be difficult to know for sure. Until then, the danger of communal alienation remains a real one and concrete images of redemption elusive.

29 Trible challenges Hagar's liberation in her analysis of the two departures into the wilderness. She remarks that language in the two departures mirrors the language used to describe the Exodus story, in which Pharaoh casts out the Israelites from Egypt, destining them for a wilderness sojourn. However,

whereas God sides with the Israelites in the Exodus, God does not ultimately advocate for the Egyptian woman in her exodus from the biblical patriarch. Trible also argues that in the second departure, God does not fulfill the promise of Hagar's descendants, but rather, this is a promise that Hagar must ensure for herself when she procures a bride for Ishmael from Egypt. Hagar therefore poses a theological challenge to the modern reader because of the contrast between a God who ultimately liberates Israel but does not appear to liberate Hagar. Summarily, Trible concludes that, "Hagar is Israel, from exodus to exile, yet with differences. And those differences yield terror. All who are heirs of Sarah and Abraham, by flesh and spirit, must answer for the terror in Hagar's story. To neglect the theological challenge she presents is to falsify faith." Trible, *Texts of Terror*, 22–29.

30 For an analysis of the pastoral use of refraining from theodicy and instead asking the question "What now?" in the aftermath of suffering, see John Swinton, *Raging with Compassion: Pastoral Responses to the Problem of Evil* (London: SCM Press, 2018).

31 One could read this argument in a way that supports continued abuse—how is, for instance, such a reading any different than telling a woman in an abusive relationship to return to her abuser and leave another time? That is not the intent of this argument. For instance, it is not the intent of this reading to argue that God allowed Hagar to return to Sarah and Abraham in the first departure in order to continue her abuse but rather to facilitate her survival and Ishmael's and, once facilitated, to then allow Hagar and Ishmael to depart for the second time for the purpose of gaining ultimate freedom. However, one might still respond that it would have been more ideal for God to facilitate Hagar's survival during her first departure. A potential response could come from best possible worlds arguments; however, in such a scenario as this, the philosophical exercise maintains a degree of futility. Instead, the "What now?" question might resonate more—given that Hagar was raped and is with child, what is necessary for her survival and her long-term liberation? In such a scenario, it may be that in the short term what was necessary was for Hagar to have the protection of the tribe as she birthed her son and then to regain strength for the wilderness journey to follow. This is not to intimate that it is better for the abused woman to stay with her abuser; however, it is to say that the abused woman will have a much harder time leaving if she does not know the location of a domestic violence shelter or have a penny saved. Immediate freedom might be preferable, but process may need to occur in order to achieve her long-term liberation.

32 For an in-depth analysis of Genie's linguistic development and how the development of language relates to the development of self-concept, see Susan Curtiss, *Genie: A Psycholinguistic Study of a Modern-Day "Wild Child"* (New York: Academic Press, 1977).

33 Martin Luther—at first an unlikely conversation partner, given the others cited—reflects on the theological significance of time in regards to healing from reproductive loss when he writes, "God is not angry with them [mothers] or with others who are involved. This is a test to develop patience." Luther's theology of suffering differs from what I propose. I am not saying that the purpose of suffering for the surrogate or any other participant in assisted reproduction is for the purpose of teaching lessons from the divine that, presumably, could not be taught in a less painful way, thereby providing a justification for the problem of evil. Such a theology discounts the possibility that the suffering experienced may outweigh goods learned through patience. This problem is intensified if the culmination of patience does not occur during this mortal life, thereby raising the question of the goodness of premortem existence on the whole.

Instead, I propose not so much a reason for surrogate suffering as a response to a potential kind of suffering–namely, divine-human alienation in which alienation is essentially the disconnection of process from time. In such a proposal, progress does not occur because process cannot occur, and time appears static as a result. Alienation can be addressed through the reintegration of time and process; this reintegration may not culminate in the premortem life, for process itself is ongoing. Such a proposal does not presume to address *why* evil or suffering occur; rather, it seeks to define what one form of evil or suffering is—alienation—and what an appropriate response to that form looks like.

See Martin Luther, "Comfort for Women Who Have Had a Miscarriage," trans. James Raun, in Frantz and Stimming, *Hope Deferred*, 67–70. For a pastoral theology of evil that discards the question of "why" in favor of the question of "What now?" see Swinton, *Raging with Compassion*. For further pastoral reflections on the nature of time and its intersection with theology and disability studies, see John Swinton, *Becoming Friends of Time: Disability, Timefullness, and Gentle Discipleship* (Waco, Tex.: Baylor University Press, 2017).

34 Research into the prevalence of anonymous surrogacy has been scant. However, more has been done to research anonymous gamete donation, perhaps because of its prevalence in the United States, if not elsewhere. Most gamete donors remain anonymous in the United States, though most clinics offer the option of known-donor procedures. Michelle L. McGowan and Leah Wilson and William D. Petok suggest that anonymous gamete donation tends to be the norm in the United States for a variety of reasons including a desire to maintain secrecy about the child's genetic origins and an interest in protecting the donor's privacy. Yet while medical professionals in the United States—where a majority of gamete donations remain anonymous—generally accept these reasons for anonymous donation, they are less commonly accepted in Oceania and Europe, where several countries have implemented laws

outlawing anonymous donation on the grounds that children deserve access to their genetic origins. See McGowan and Wilson, "Oocyte Donation," in Goldfarb, *Third-Party Reproduction*, 55. See also Petok, "Sperm Donation," in Goldfarb, *Third-Party Reproduction*, 162.

35 Parents may choose to not to disclose a child's origin for a variety of reasons, including privacy concerns and fears that the lack of a genetic relationship would upset the child or threaten the identity of the parents, that a lack of genetic information about a donor would upset the child, that the knowledge would disrupt relationships between the parents and the child, or that the information is irrelevant because parenthood is a social contract and not a biological one. It may also arise because of parents' own cognitions about the third party. Writing about embryo donation—a technology whereby intended parents donate unused embryos from a previous procedure, thereby resulting in a child from donated egg and sperm—social scientists in the United Kingdom found that parents rarely thought about or talked about the donors with their spouse. See MacCallum, "Embryo Donation Parents' Attitudes," 517–23.

36 Intriguingly, studies have also found that children conceived via gamete donation are less likely to be told of their origins than children brought into a family via adoption. However, like the trajectory of adoption—where disclosure rates were historically low but have been recently on the rise—it is becoming more common for American parents to disclose third-party use. There has also been minimal research into embryo donation, which would be genetically akin to adoption. Childress-Beatty, "Embryo Donation," 116–17.

37 Amanda J. Turner and Adrian Coyle found that teenagers and adults who discovered that they were conceived with donated genetic material experienced a number of detrimental cognitions and feelings, including mistrust, abandonment by medical professionals who advocated nondisclosure, and a sense of frustration or loss that they could not obtain donor information. In regard to this final issue, writing on the legal aspects of sperm donation, Stephanie O. Corley and Maxwell Mehlman explain that "children conceived with the use of anonymous sperm are likened to adoptive children, and studies have shown that insecurities arise in adoptees because of the lack of information about the child's biological parent(s)." Turner and Coyle therefore suggest that individuals told later about the involvement of a third party subsequently experience themselves as different from the family who raised them. Reinforcing this data, Petok explains that children of sperm donors who discover the use of the donor later in life "can experience a disruption of identity. In essence, they are not the persons they assumed they were." As a result, he argues that "openness produces better psychological results for children conceived with donor sperm and for the families in which they are raised." One might make similar arguments for other types of third-party involvement, including surrogacy. See Turner and Coyle, "What Does It Mean to Be a

Donor Offspring?" 2041–51; Corley and Mehlman, "Sperm Donation," 154; and Petok, "Sperm Donation," in Goldfarb, *Third-Party Reproduction*, 165.

38 Given current medical technology and the desire of children to access their origins, the possibility that donors and surrogates can retain anonymity into the future may be decreasing with the advent of websites that track DNA, including sites such as the Donor Sibling Registry—which allows children of donors to use their DNA to find half-siblings who share the same donor—and Family Tree DNA, a site that helps individuals locate biological relatives. These websites not only allow children to find half-siblings, but also help children locate their egg or sperm donor. Intriguingly, then, the community of children birthed via third-party reproduction is using the "third space" of the internet to exert agency in order to learn more about their identity when other means fail. See Susan L. Crockin and Lauren M. Nussbaum, "Embryo Donation: Legal Aspects," in Goldfarb, *Third-Party Reproduction*, 105. For examples of children of donors who have used sites like these to locate their donors, see Rachel Lehmann-Haupt, "Are Sperm Donors Really Anonymous Anymore? DNA Testing Makes Them Easy to Trace," *Slate*, March 1, 2010, http://www.slate.com/articles/double_x/doublex/2010/02/are_sperm_donors_really_anonymous_anymore.html. See also Mary Harris, "Lost Then Found," *On the Media*, National Public Radio, October 18, 2013, http://www.onthemedia.org/story/lost-then-found/transcript/. For more on the possibility of anonymous sperm donors being discovered in film, see *Delivery Man*, a film directed by Ken Scott (New York: DreamWorks, 2013); and *Starbuck*, a film directed by Ken Scott (Montreal: Caramel Films, 2011). See also *The Kids Are All Right*, a film directed by Lisa Cholodenko (Los Angeles: Focus Features, 2010).

5 Consonant Dependency Care as a New Vision for Family

1 By way of example, the Roman Catholic Church describes the family as a "domestic church," wherein procreation mirrors God's creative abilities and through which "faith, hope and charity" can be practiced in such a way as to cause the family to be the "original cell of social life." The Church of Jesus Christ of Latter Day Saints likewise believes that family is the fundamental unit of society, while Anglican theologian Frederick Dennison Maurice argues not only that God can be known through human relationships but also that familial relationships provide the most intimate way of gaining that knowledge. See Catholic Church, *Catechism of the Catholic Church: Revised in Accordance with the Official Latin Text Promulgated by Pope John Paul II* (Vatican City: Libreria Editrice Vaticana, 1997), part 3, section 2, chapter 2, article 4, I.2204–2206; II.2207, http://www.vatican.va/archive/ccc_css/archive/catechism/p3s2c2a4.htm. See also Frederick Dennison Maurice, *To Build Christ's Kingdom: F. D. Maurice and His Writings* (London: Canterbury Press Norwich, 2007).

2 For a critique of equality as sameness, see Eva Feder Kittay, *Love's Labor: Essays on Women, Equality, and Dependency* (New York: Routledge, 1999).

3 One could make the case that a desire for biological connection is implicit in adoption practices as well, specifically in the desire of parents to adopt children that most closely resemble themselves. That tendency has economic overtones that result in racial implications: those with white skin, who possess a majority of the wealth in the United States, are more likely to have the means to adopt, and because they often prefer white babies, such infants become a desired commodity while darker-skinned infants become easier to obtain but less desirable.

4 This is not to say that third-party reproduction can never be discerned as the desired ending to one's reproductive story, but it is to say that this desire has the right to be discerned without undue influence from external sources.

5 Though it is not primarily focused on third-party reproduction, for an extensive analysis of the way that Protestant culture constrained and determined the narrative reproductive freedom of American individuals in the twentieth century generally, see Amy Laura Hall, *Conceiving Parenthood: American Protestantism and the Spirit of Reproduction* (Grand Rapids: Eerdmans, 2008).

6 This understanding of the self supposes that the self does not construct itself autonomously and then relate to other selves but that construction occurs through relationships with other selves, thereby affiliating it with relational understandings of the self often proposed by feminist philosophers. For more on feminist philosophical visions of the relational self, see Susan Brison, "Personal Identity and Relational Selves" in *The Routledge Companion to Feminist Philosophy*, ed. Ann Garry, Serene J. Khader, and Alison Stone (Basingstoke, UK: Taylor & Francis, 2017), 218–30; Lorraine Code, "Second Persons," in *What Can She Know? Feminist Theory and the Construction of Knowledge* (Ithaca, N.Y.: Cornell University Press, 1991), 71–109; and Diana T. Meyers, ed., *Feminists Rethink the Self* (Boulder, Colo.: Westview Press, 1997). For an interesting analysis of the relational self as it relates to contract theory, justice, and nurturing, see Seyla Benhabib, "The Generalized and the Concrete Other: The Kohlberg-Gilligan Controversy and Moral Theory," in *Women and Moral Theory*, ed. Eva Feder Kittay and Diana T. Meyers (Lanham, Md.: Rowman & Littlefield, 1987), 154–77.

7 For more on the psychological effects of stigmatization on women who suffer from infertility, see Arthur L. Greil, "Infertility and Psychological Distress: A Review of the Literature," *Social Science and Medicine* 45, no. 11 (1997): 1679–704; and Arthur L. Greil, Kathleen Slauson-Blevins, and Julia McQuillan, "The Experience of Infertility: A Review of Recent Literature," *Sociology of Health & Illness* 32, no. 1 (2010): 140–62.

8 Foster parenthood also requires such evaluation, though these are assumed to be short-term placements, except in situations where fostering leads to adoption.

9 Kittay, *Love's Labor,* 16.

10 Economic structures related to elder care in the United States might serve as a case study in this regard. Many adults rely on children for care in their old age, both because of the comfort children provide and because of economic constraints—while it is costly to hire an aide or nurse, a child can function as a dependency worker who provides the same care free of cost. In this way, care of the elderly remains within the boundaries of the family so that the family unit maintains a degree of autonomy. In contrast, those without children face economic challenges related to their care in old age that those with children may find mitigated in some ways. One could make the argument that those without children may be more likely to be financially stable and have more to spend on their own care in later life because they did not have to spend as much on child-related expenses during their prime earning years. Even so, the tacit societal expectation that children will provide at least some care to their elderly parents in the United States offers those with children a good that those without children do not have. Invoking Kittay, one wonders what the transformative practice might be here. What might society be like, for instance, if *all* elderly individuals in need received consistent and meaningful support from not only biological family but also from their neighbors and societal structures designed to assist with their physical and psychological needs? Indeed, this would provide for the needs of those without children while simultaneously providing some respite for those children who function as dependency workers for their elderly parents and who often sacrifice their own needs in order to do so.

11 Peggy Orenstein documents the way that medical professionals can use their power to exploit intended parents' hopes. She suggests that some adults want to have children so much that they can become addicted to hope and, subsequently, become subject to exploitation by medical professionals who know how to manipulate that hope. See Orenstein, *Waiting for Daisy.*

12 For an extensive theological and historical analysis of family from a Christian perspective, see Lisa Sowle Cahill, *Family: A Christian Social Perspective* (Minneapolis: Fortress, 2000). For a practical theological analysis of family that specifically engages gender roles, see Bonnie Miller-McLemore, *Also a Mother: Work and Family as Theological Dilemma* (Nashville, Tenn.: Abingdon, 1994). For multidisciplinary theological analysis of family—including perspectives from practical theology and history—see Don S. Browning et al., *From Culture Wars to Common Ground: Religion and the American Family Debate* (Louisville: Westminster John Knox, 1997).

13 Eva Kittay problematizes the notion that justice can be described in terms of equality by taking issue with the reference classes that serve as norms for equality. To be equal, Kittay argues, is for a nondominant class to seek identicality with the reference class in significant ways; however, when the reference class itself is problematic, then seeking to become synonymous with it

does not ensure a just outcome so much as it obtains the privilege afforded to the reference class. Kittay, *Love's Labor,* 6–7.

14 Having proposed that the family is primarily a unit of social belonging, one might find it worthwhile to recall the question "What is the context for asking what the family is?" In this case, the question is being answered within the context of culture in the United States. In contrast, Rahul Sharma embarks upon the task of redefining the family from an Indian perspective, while noting that *family* has no uniform definition across culture or across academic discipline; even the censuses of different countries define the family different ways depending on what kind of data they seek. Sharma also intriguingly expands the use of *nuclear* as a metaphor in relation to the family to consider the proton, electron, atom, or molecular equivalent of families. See Rahul Sharma, "The Family and Family Structure Classification Redefined for the Current Times," *Journal of Family Medicine and Primary Care* 2, no. 4 (2013): 306–10.

15 For a selection of liberal ethical and philosophical perspectives on surrogacy, see Richard J. Arneson, "Commodification and Commercial Surrogacy," *Philosophy and Public Affairs* 21 (1992): 132–64; H. M. Malm, "Paid Surrogacy: Arguments and Responses," *Public Affairs Quarterly* 3 (1989): 57–66; and John A. Robertson, *Children of Choice: Freedom and the New Reproductive Technologies* (Princeton, N.J.: Princeton University Press, 1994).

16 Jennifer A. Parks references the well-publicized Baby Manji surrogacy case to parse what is at stake in these two perspectives. Baby Manji was born to an Indian surrogate in Anand in 2008, culminating a contract with a Japanese couple. However, the couple—the Yamadas—divorced prior to Baby Manji's birth, and the intended mother stated that she no longer desired the baby following the separation. The Indian surrogate, who never claimed to want the baby in the first place, also declined custody of the child. Meanwhile, the intended father was unable to claim Baby Manji because Indian law requires that a child's passport only be issued in conjunction with the mother's. Baby Manji was eventually issued a Japanese passport and allowed to depart for Japan after her paternal grandmother traveled to India and asked for custody of the child. Parks analyzes the Baby Manji episode from the perspective of both liberalism and care ethics, noting, "Liberal theory cannot address the narrative and relational harm to which Manji was subjected. Not only were her rights to citizenship under threat (something a straightforwardly liberal argument *can* account for), but so was her right to be cared for, to be an individual of particular concern. . . . In an important way, without people to whom Baby Manji is special, unique, and loved, she does not exist—an assertion that is true for every human being everywhere in the world." See Jennifer A. Parks, "Care Ethics and the Global Practice of Commercial Surrogacy," *Bioethics* 24 no. 7 (2010): 335.

17 Eva Kittay references the experiences of women to exemplify the difficulties with correlating sameness and equality. Women often desire the kind of equality that grants them the same rights given to men—the right to own land, inherit money, vote, wear pants, work, or receive equal pay in that workplace. Such practices allow women to approach the norm of the male reference class, but these practices do not necessarily result in equality, and indeed, Kittay suggests that granting women such sameness does not in and of itself result in equality because of the dependency demands for which women find themselves responsible by virtue of either biology or culture. Care of infants, children, and the elderly all traditionally fall to women in such a pervasive way, Kittay argues, that it "has thrown doubt on the aspiration that they will ever share the world with men in equality." Kittay, *Love's Labor,* 16.

18 Kittay, *Love's Labor,* 16.

19 Per the latter point, Kittay writes that women's frequent engagement with dependency work allows them to see the inevitable connections that exist between humans both for good and for ill. She writes, "Members of human communities are engaged in interdependencies. They emphasize the fact that the independent individual is always a fictive creation of those men sufficiently privileged to shift the concern for dependence onto others. Understandings of equality that remain based in the independence of individuals, whether they call for equality simpliciter or sex equality, will also exclude as they include." Kittay, *Love's Labor,* 17.

20 Here Kittay invokes the work of Carol Gilligan to offer a new vision for equality and justice: Gilligan describes a scene where a young boy wants to play pirates, while a young girl wants to play neighbors. The approach from traditional notions of equality would be to set a timer and tell the children that they can play neighbors for half the time and then pirates for the other half. However, the girl suggests what Gilligan calls an "inclusive" approach to the problem instead, suggesting that they play a new game in which the pirates are neighbors. Kittay concludes that it is such inclusive visions that offer the greatest potential to resolve matters of inequality between dependency workers and other groups precisely because it calls for an imaginative approach that dismantles the supremacy of sameness. Kittay, *Love's Labor,* 239.

21 Kittay, *Love's Labor,* 181.

22 Kittay, *Love's Labor,* 181.

23 Kittay, *Love's Labor,* 38.

24 Kittay, *Love's Labor,* 181. Kittay notes that dependency work in this extended sense involves tasks historically delegated to women.

25 What Kittay terms the "extended model of dependency care" in some ways bears resemblance to what Delores Williams calls "social-role surrogacy," a type of surrogacy that occurs when a black woman takes onto herself responsibilities that usually belong to someone else despite her desire not to do so. Williams offers the role of mammy as a historic example, explaining that

the mammy took responsibility for domestic affairs of the house that were traditionally assumed by the plantation owner's wife, responsibilities such as looking after children and supervising housekeeping. Williams argues that both biological and social-role surrogacy take place in the lives of the antebellum and post-antebellum African American women, and with reference to social-role surrogacy, Williams distinguishes between the two periods, employing the term "coerced surrogacy" to refer to social-role surrogacy during slavery and "voluntary surrogacy" to refer to social-role surrogacy after it. Having stated their similarities, however, Kittay's vision of extended dependency care does not seem to rely upon coercion of the worker; theoretically, the extended dependency worker *could* choose to do something else. Additionally, Kittay does not make race a central point of discussion in her work of extended dependency workers in the way that grounds the womanist study Williams undertakes. Williams, *Sisters in the Wilderness*, 60–67.

26 Social scientists query at length whether the surrogate is best conceived as a type of mother or a type of worker. Pande notes a similar conversation surrounds analysis of sex workers, for both sex workers and surrogates undertake responsibilities that most traditionally fall within the sphere of a woman's responsibilities within marriage, in other words, that belong to a wife. The wife, as spouse, does not get paid to either have sex with her husband or carry children; rather, both are conceived as her role within the marriage relationship. However, when women adopt these responsibilities professionally, outside of marriage, then it problematizes assumptions about the appropriateness of commodifying such an act. Pande, *Wombs in Labor,* 64–84.

27 Carmel Shalev proposes that liberal approaches to surrogacy justify "need" language by predicating themselves on autonomy, freedom, individual liberty, and gains that outweigh harms. These justify the development of a free-market economy for assisted reproduction. As she explains the logic: third-party assisted reproduction becomes permissible if one person wants to buy the reproductive services of another and the other person wants to sell those services, for both freely offer themselves and both experience a net gain. Shalev critiques this argument on the grounds that freedom in actuality functions as a convenient justification for profit and greed because "novel reproductive technologies create new markets of consumers. . . . Once a new market is established, the greed of medical entrepreneurs is complemented by a consumerist discourse of desire. The language of 'would like' or 'want' translates to 'need,' which then turns into a sense of entitlement (to have a child) and the assertion of a 'right' (to use the technology), together with a demand for immediate gratification." See Carmel Shalev, "An Ethic of Care and Responsibility: Reflections on Third-Party Reproduction," *Medical Studies* 3 no. 3 (2012): 1501–51.

28 To that end, Shalev observes that intended parents who use any form of third-party reproduction, particularly women, obtain their desire for parenthood

"at substantial cost to other women who assist them in doing so. For each of the ten times that one woman seeks an egg donation, there is another woman who has placed herself at great risk to give her what she wants." Shalev, "Ethics of Care and Responsibility," 149.

29 Pregnancy is not covered under the Americans with Disabilities Act but may be treated as a temporary disability. Accommodations are required per the Pregnancy Discrimination Act, which is an amendment to Title VII and the Family and Medical Leave Act.

30 Institute of Health Metrics and Evaluations, "Maternal Mortality Ratio," Data Visualizations, https://vizhub.healthdata.org/sdg/, accessed November 4, 2017.

31 Black women, in particular, find themselves particularly affected, as this population is more likely to suffer from obesity and its medical complications. However, this does not in and of itself account for the maternal mortality rate in the United States, which maintains its status as the worst among industrialized nations even if only white women are subject to analysis. Sabrina Tavernise, "Maternal Mortality Rate in U.S. Rises, Defying Global Trendy, Study Finds," *New York Times*, September 21, 2016.

32 As of 2017, 6 percent of block grants for "maternal and child health" go to women who give birth under the Title V Maternal and Child Health Services Block Grant Program. Julia Belluz, "California Decided It Was Tired of Women Bleeding to Death in Childbirth," *Vox*, June 29, 2017.

33 Analysis shows that errors in data collection contributed to Texas's high maternal mortality rate. However, even accounting for these errors, the United States languishes behind many of its peers when it comes to maternal mortality outcomes. See Sonia Baeva et al., "Identifying Maternal Deaths in Texas Using an Enhanced Method, 2012," *Obstetrics and Gynecology* 131, no. 5 (April 8, 2018): 762–69. See also Meagan Flynn, "Texas's Maternal Mortality Rate Was Unbelievably High. Now We Know Why," *Washington Post*, April 11, 2018.

34 Placenta percreta, increta, and accreta develop primarily in women who have had C-sections prior; they are uncommon in women who have never had children or only had vaginal births. Risk increases with the number of C-sections a woman has, primarily due to scarring from the surgery. See "Placenta Accreta," American Pregnancy Association, October 19, 2018, http://americanpregnancy.org/pregnancy-complications/placenta-accreta/.

35 California implemented a policy requiring that such hemorrhage kits be nearby during labor and delivery; consequently, the state has a maternal mortality rate approximately three times lower than the national average. Summarily, Eugene Declercq states that "the argument we make internationally is that [a high maternal death rate] is often a reflection of how society views women. . . . In other countries, we worry about the culture—women are not particularly valued, so they don't set up systems to care for them at all. I

think we have a similar problem in the U.S." Eugene Declercq, qtd., Belluz, "California decided."

36 Here I differ from Parks, who places surrogates in a necessarily subservient position to intended parents because of the latter's wealth and power. In contrast, I argue that while the surrogate may be subservient in regard to financial resources, she is in a position of power due to her fertility such that she can simultaneously be under threat of exploitation and also be the threat for exploitation of intended parents. Parks, "Care Ethics," 339.

37 Susan Wendell observes that the pace and structure of modern life contributes to the construction of disability. In relation to reproductive difficulties, one could argue that the pacing and structure of the United States encourages adults to forgo childbearing in order to attain socially desirable—even necessary—goods, including an education and stable career. Moreover, there are negative societal consequences for those who reproduce at an early age, as evidenced by the stigmatization of teenage mothers. As a result, adults face more reproductive difficulties because they embark upon childbearing at a later age; were society structured differently in its value of the procreative body, then perhaps rates of reproductive difficulties would decrease because the timing of reproduction would change. For more on the social construction of disability and its relationship to the pace and structure of life in the United States, see Susan Wendell, *The Rejected Body: Feminist Philosophical Reflections on Disability* (New York: Routledge, 1996), 11–35. For more on the social construction of disability as it specifically relates to infertility, see Moss and Baden, *Reconceiving Infertility*, 1–20. For an overview of different medical definitions of disability and how they relate to infertility, see Abha Khetarpal and Satendra Singh, "Infertility: Why Can't We Classify This Inability as Disability?" *Australiasian Medical Journal* 5, no. 6 (2012): 334–39.

38 While these programs illustrate the assumption that adults in the United States will reproduce, it is interesting to note that all of these programs value reproduction because it produces workers, not because it produces individuals with whom relationships might be cultivated, thus implying that the United States places instrumental and not intrinsic value on the humans created through reproduction. Indeed, those programs that supposedly should value the reproductive adult or the child birthed by her seem to consistently be targeted or under threat of losing funding. Such structures include Medicaid for coverage of pregnant and postpartum women, Child Protective Services, and public education.

39 Kittay suggests that construction ends when mutuality ends because sometimes one person is necessarily dependent on another rather than being dependent through construction. To that end she writes that visions of interdependency reach their limits when such situations arise: "While the image of a mutuality and interdependence among persons is an important one . . . there are moments when we are not 'inter'dependent. We are simply dependent and

cannot reciprocate. If you have a fever of 105, the dependence you have is not socially constructed." Kittay, *Love's Labor,* 180.

40 As a potential counter to this argument, Swedish researchers found that Swedish couples who employed Indian surrogates—domestic surrogacy in Sweden is illegal—simultaneously felt that the money they paid to surrogates bettered their lives while also sensing that Indian surrogacy was poorly regulated and that Sweden ought to allow for surrogacy so as to create healthier regulative structures. In this way, the Swedish parent's advocacy may be said to function as a kind of care-based relationship, even if the Swedish parent never met the surrogate, which was not necessarily the case. See Anna Arvidsson, Sarah Johnsdotter, and Birgitta Essén, "Views of Swedish Commisioning Parents Relating to the Exploitation Discourse in Using Transnational Surrogacy," *PLOS ONE* 10, no. 5 (2015): 1–12.

41 Connected vulnerability harkens back to one of the central tenets of care ethics, that humans are necessarily in relationship with one another and often connected through vulnerability. Openness and responsiveness within the contexts of known relationships therefore become central to acknowledging that connection, such that practices of anonymity counter it. See Patricia Bender, "A Dialogue between Virtue Ethics and Care Ethics," *Theoretical Medicine* 18 (1997): 47–61.

42 Shalev uses the broader framework of care ethics to make a similar argument specifically concerning the women who participate in surrogacy—namely, the intended mother and surrogate herself. Shalev notes that each is dependent on the other and vulnerable to the other for needs to be met; as a result, the relationship that necessarily exists between the women leads to each woman having a responsibility toward the other. Proximity is therefore necessary for responsibility to manifest. Shalev, "An Ethic of Care and Responsibility," 154.

Conclusion: Generalized Surrogacy and a Global Family

1 In her own words: "One thing is certain. Surrogacy has been a negative force in African-American women's lives. It has been used by both men and women of the ruling class, as well as by some black men, to keep black women in the service of other people's needs and goals." Williams, *Sisters in the Wilderness*, 81. Catherine Keller offers an alternate reading of Williams when she writes that "Williams cannot in these terms simply reject surrogacy as evil; it is the imposition of surrogacy and its injustices that she rejects." Keller, "Delores Williams," 90. Keller here seems to be extrapolating Williams' interpretation of the Hagar story to her conclusions about surrogacy on the whole without considering her reading of coerced and voluntary surrogacy in the lives of black women; it is furthermore worth noting that Keller is primarily concerned with how Williams' reading affects her theology of the cross. To that end, one might critique Keller for only considering one part of Williams' interpretation of surrogacy in her discussion. For an alternate interpretation, see Dianne M. Stewart, "Womanist God-Talk on the Cutting Edge of Theology and Black

Religious Studies: Assessing the Contribution of Delores Williams," *Union Seminary Quarterly Review*, 58, nos. 3–4 (Fall 2004): 69–74.

2 Williams, *Sisters in the Wilderness*, 67.

3 Theoretically, the possibility also exists for one person to be both Person A and Person B. Monica Coleman, for example, proposes that a woman who suffers a miscarriage or abortion is both surrogate and mother because she is pregnant with but does not raise the child she carries (making her a surrogate), and yet she understands herself as having a maternal identity toward that particular fetus and cared for it as such. See Coleman, *Making a Way Out of No Way: A Womanist Theology*, Innovations: African American Religious Thought (Minneapolis: Fortress, 2008), 206.

4 Marilyn McCord Adams makes an intriguing argument that Christ's human nature participated in these forms of cultural misorientation during his life, namely those collective evils that society did not acknowledge as sinful. If this is the case, then God gains embodied understanding of the experiences of Person B. *Christ and Horrors: The Coherence of Christology* (Cambridge: Cambridge University Press, 2008), 80–144.

5 James Gilligan proposes that the prison system distributes shame and guilt in the prison population in such a way that prisoners become scapegoats both inside the prison's power structures and as a class in relation to society at large. Gilligan argues that the perpetuation of shame—which in turn leads to violence—has become an essential way for Americans in positions of power to maintain their power. By causing certain subsets of individuals in the United States to be likely to experience shame in their everyday lives, violence continues and perpetuates, thereby keeping these individuals in a state of subservience. See James Gilligan, *Violence: Reflections on a National Epidemic* (New York: Vintage Books, 1997).

6 This aligns with how Delores Williams understands social-role surrogacy. From the perspective of a different discipline, Susan Brison also writes about how sexual assault and rape require self-reconstruction on the part of survivors after the event. See both *Sisters in the Wilderness* and *Aftermath*.

7 Pitkin argues that power-to-do involves the ability not just to exact agency but also the potential or capacity to exact agency. Such a definition aligns with chapter one's conception of agency as not just successful completion of the agential act but rather the ability to attempt to enact agency if the individual desires to do so. For contrasting views of power as power-over vs. power-to-do, see Robert A. Dahl, "The Concept of Power," *Behavioral Science* 2, no. 3 (2007): 1–15; and Hanna F. Pitkin, *Wittgenstein and Justice: On the Significance of Ludwig Wittgenstein for Social and Political Thought* (Berkeley: University of Berkeley Press, 1993), 276.

8 Judith Butler makes a corollary argument concerning gender construction, arguing—via Foucault—that women (Person B) exist in systems of male (Person A) subjectivity such that "the feminist subject turns out to be discursively

constituted by the very political system that is supposed to facilitate its emancipation." See Judith Butler, *Gender Trouble: Feminism and the Subversion of Identity* (New York: Routledge, 2015), 2-3.

9 Social psychological research findings reinforce what is known as the proximity principle, which states that proximity is essential to the initial creation of relationships. To that end, Festinger, Schachter and Bach studied a dormitory at Massachusetts Institute of Technology and found that friendships were most likely to develop between individuals housed on the same floor, except in situations where individuals lived either near mailboxes, which members of both floors visited regularly, or near stairs, which also resulted in a greater frequency of exposure to members of other floors. Contemporary studies appear to reinforce this finding. Preciado et al. found that proximity played a role in the formation of friendships in teenagers in a rural Swedish town, while Amichai-Hamburger, Kingsbury, and Schneider found that internet-based interactions were more likely to occur between individuals who lived in the same geographical area and who had preexisting relationships than those who did not. See L. Festinger, S. Schachter, and K. Bach, *Social Pressures in Informal Groups* (Stanford, Calif.: Stanford University Press, 1963). See also P. Preciado, T. Snijders, W. J. Burk, H. Stattin, and M. Kerr, "Does Proximity Matter? Distance Dependence of Adolescent Friendships," *Social Networks* 34, no. 1 (2011): 18–31; and Y. Amichai-Hamburger, M. Kingsbury, and B. H. Schneider, "Friendship: An Old Concept with a New Meaning?" *Computers in Human Behavior* 29, no. 1 (2012): 33–39.

10 See Beverley Ann Fehr, *Friendship Processes* (Thousand Oaks, Calif.: Sage, 1999), 13–15.

11 Carolyn Weisz and Lisa F. Wood's research on what creates "best friends" uncovered that "social-identity support" separated best friends from other forms of relationship. Individuals were most likely to think of another person as his or her "best friend" if that individual supported the individual's perception of his or her most fundamental identity characteristics. Hence, a man who most wanted to be known as a Christian would most value a friend who characterized him as such, while a person who most wanted to be known as a mother would most value a friend who saw her that way. Often these best friends maintained social-identity support by participating in the same groups that helped them establish the identities they sought for themselves; other times, the best friend was outside of the group that the individual sought to identify with but still affirmative of that individual's role. These findings held across genders. See Carolyn Weisz and Lisa F. Wood, "Social Identity Support and Friendship Outcomes: A Longitudinal Study Predicting Who Will Be Friends and Best Friends Four Years Later," *Journal of Personal and Social Relationships* 22, no. 3 (2005): 416–32. Weisz also found that self-identification with a given group may determine behavioral outcomes, as demonstrated by her study on addiction, which found that when individuals identified with

a group whose beliefs or characteristics contradicted alcohol or cocaine use, they were more likely to be abstinent at the three-month mark. See Carolyn Weisz, "Social Identities and Response to Treatment for Alcohol and Cocaine Abuse," *Addictive Behaviors* 21, no. 4 (1996): 445–58.

12 Weisz, "Social Identity Support and Friendship Outcomes," 416–32.

13 This depiction of friendship as mutual self-enhancing generalized surrogacy might appear to challenge reciprocity. Per Aristotle's categorizations of friendship as based in pleasure, utility, or virtue, social-identity support would initially seem to indicate that utility grounds friendship because of the way that Friend A validates self-concept through the support given by Friend B. Friend B therefore provides utility to Friend A that Friend A values, and vice versa. Likewise, one could argue that social-identity support suggests that friendship is rooted in pleasure because Friend A derives pleasure from Friend B's reinforcement of Friend A's desired self. In either case, any reciprocity that exists is based not in concern for the other but in what that utility or pleasure affords the individual, such that Friend A is primarily friends with Friend B because of the benefits that exist for Friend A and vice versa.

Such an interpretation would be reductive. Indeed, Friends A and B provide utility and pleasure to one another, but they do so because of a shared commitment to social-identity support. In other words, Friend B provides the same kind of support to Friend A, and both Friend A and Friend B agree that such support is of value. This kind of reciprocity suggests that Friends A and B share a belief that cultivating self-concept is important, and so the friends value one another not just because of the actions they take or the pleasure they derive from them but because of the beliefs they mutually inhabit. As a result, Friend B values Friend A for his or her virtuous character, thereby suggesting that social-identity support friendship functions more as a virtue-oriented friendship than as a utility or pleasure-based one. Social psychological findings about the general lack of value afforded utility in friendship further supports this assertion. See Fehr, *Friendship Processes,* 13–15.

14 The extent to which a given society accepts negative projected desire as cultural misorientation might be said to be a form of original sin, where original sin is defined as the transmission of and tacit acceptance of such normed values.

15 Michael Banner proposes that the Gospel stories do not propose the eradication of biological kinship but rather a reconfiguration of it: "Brothers aren't banished from the New Testament but reappear as brothers of all within the community of believers . . . This is not, then, an unkinning, but a rekinning—even if the reappropriation establishes what should be regarded as, in the case of the community of discipleship, a 'counter-cultural social structure.'" Michael C. Banner, *The Ethics of Everyday Life: Moral Theology, Social Anthropology, and the Imagination of the Human* (Oxford: Oxford University Press, 2016), 42–43.

16 Banner, *Ethics of Everyday Life*, 59.

17 Williams would most certainly take issue with the claim that surrogates address theodicy in a positive way, given her assertion that nothing salvific or positive comes from the experience of surrogacy. Presenting Jesus as the ultimate surrogate who suffers on the cross, she goes so far as to argue that Jesus' sacrifice is of essentially negative value and salvation occurs only at the resurrection. Whether Jesus' time on the cross qualifies as self-enhancing surrogacy is beyond the bounds of this project. What the assertion above intends, however, is simply to say that surrogacy can be of positive transformative value if certain preconditions exist to support its implementation as such.

18 Herman, *Trauma and Recovery*, 51–74, 133–214.

19 Banner, *Ethics of Everyday Life*, 59.

20 For an expansive historic overview of how legal structures perpetuate structures that allow for systemic racism, see Kelly Brown Douglas, *Stand Your Ground: Black Bodies and the Justice of God* (Maryknoll, N.Y.: Orbis, 2015).

Bibliography

Adams, Marilyn McCord. "Friendliness, Divine and Human." In *Rethinking the Medieval Legacy for Contemporary Theology*, edited by Anselm K. Min, 43–71. Notre Dame, Ind.: University of Notre Dame: 2014.

———. *Horrendous Evils and the Goodness of* God. Ithaca, N.Y.: Cornell University Press, 1999.

———. *Christ and Horrors: The Coherence of Christology*. Cambridge: Cambridge University Press, 2008.

Albertyn, Tertia Loebenberg. *So Close: Infertile and Addicted to Hope*. Chatham, Mich.: Porcupine Press, 2009.

American Psychiatric Association. *Diagnostic and Statistical Manual of Mental Disorders*. 5th edition (DSM-5). Washington, D.C.: American Psychiatric Publishing, 2017.

Ames, David A., and Colin B. Gracey, ed. *Good Genes? Emerging Values for Science, Religion, and Society*. Cincinnati: Forward Movement Publications, 1984.

Amichai-Hamburger, Y., M. Kingsbury, and B. H. Schneider. "Friendship: An Old Concept with a New Meaning?" *Computers in Human Behavior* 29 (2012): 33–39.

Applegarth, Linda D. "Oocyte Donation: Psychological Aspects." In Goldfarb, *Third-Party Reproduction*, 41–50.

American Pregnancy Association. "Donor Eggs." June 2012. http://www.americanpregnancy.org/infertility/donoreggs.html. Accessed June 9, 2012.

American Pregnancy Association. "Infertility." February 2012. http://americanpregnancy.org/infertility/whatisinfertility.html. Accessed June 9, 2012.

American Pregnancy Association. "Miscarriage." November 2011. http://americanpregnancy.org/pregnancycomplications/miscarriage.html. Accessed June 9, 2012.

American Pregnancy Association. "Stillbirth: Trying to Understand." January 2013. http://americanpregnancy.org/pregnancyloss/sbtryingtounderstand.html. Accessed June 9, 2012.

American Society for Reproductive Medicine. "ASRM: Frequently Asked Questions about Infertility." http://www.asrm.org/awards/index?id=3012. Accessed June 9, 2012.

Arneson, Richard J. "Commodification and Commercial Surrogacy." *Philosophy and Public Affairs* 21 (1992): 132–64.

Arvidsson, Anna, Sarah Johnsdotter, and Birgitta Essén. "Views of Swedish Commissioning Parents Relating to the Exploitation Discourse in Using Transnational Surrogacy." *PLOS ONE* 10, no. 5 (2015): 1–12.

Asch, Adrienne, and Rebecca Marmor. "Assisted Reproduction." The Hastings Center. http://www.thehastingscenter.org/Publications/BriefingBook/Detail.aspx?id=2210. Accessed June 19, 2012.

Austin, J. L. *How to Do Things with Words.* 2nd edition. Oxford: Clarendon, 2011.

Bach, Kent, and Robert M. Harnish, "Linguistic Communication and Speech Acts," *The Philosophical Review* 1 (1982).

Baker-Fletcher, Karen. *Dancing with God: The Trinity from a Womanist Perspective.* St. Louis, Mo.: Chalice, 2006.

Banner, Michael C. *The Ethics of Everyday Life: Moral Theology, Social Anthropology, and the Imagination of the Human.* Oxford: Oxford University Press, 2016.

Baeva, Sonia, Debra L. Sexton, Karen Ruggiero, Michelle L. Kormondy, Lisa M. Hollier, John Hellerstedt, Manda Hall, and Natalie P. Archer. "Identifying Maternal Deaths in Texas Using an Enhanced Method, 2012." *Obstetrics and Gynecology* 131, no. 5 (April 8, 2018): 1–8.

Baker-Fletcher, Karen. *My Sister, My Brother: Womanist and Xodus God-Talk.* Eugene, Ore.: Wipf & Stock, 2002.

Bartholet, Elizabeth. *Family Bonds: Adoption, Infertility, and the New World of Child Reproduction.* Boston: Beacon, 1999.

Bass, Dorothy, and Craig Dykstra, eds. *For Life Abundant: Practical Theology, Theological Education, and Christian Ministry.* Grand Rapids: Eerdmans, 2008.

Bauman, Tamar. "The Intergenerational Transmission of Trauma Symptoms in Children of Holocaust Survivors." PhD diss., Pace University, 2003.

Bednarowski, Mary Farrell. "New Conversations in Religion and Literature." *Arts* 1, no. 3 (1989): 4–7.

Belenky, Mary, Blythe Clinchy, Nancy Goldberger, and Jill Tarule. *Women's Ways of Knowing: The Development of Self, Voice, and Mind.* 10th anniversary ed. New York: Basic Books, 1997.

Bender, Patricia. "A Dialogue between Virtue Ethics and Care Ethics." *Theoretical Medicine* 18 (1997): 47–61.

Benhabib, Seyla. "The Generalized and the Concrete Other: The Kohlberg-Gilligan Controversy and Moral Theory." In *Women and Moral Theory*, edited by Eva Feder Kittay and Diana T. Meyers, 154–77. Lanham, Md.: Rowman & Littlefield, 1987.

Berg, B. J., J. F. Wilson, and P. J. Weingartner. "Psychological Sequelae of Infertility Treatment: The Role of Gender and Sex-Role Identification." *Social Science and Medicine* 33, no. 9 (1991): 1071–80.

Bergmann, S. "Reproductive Agency and Projects: Germans Searching for Egg Donation in Spain and the Czech Republic." *Reproductive BioMedicine Online* 23, no. 5 (2011): 600–608.

Berry, Wanda Warren. "Feminist Theology: The 'Verbing' of Ultimate/Intimate Reality in Mary Daly." In *Feminist Interpretations of Mary Daly: Re-reading the Canon*, edited by Sarah Lucia Hoagland and Marilyn Frye, 37–39. University Park, Pa.: Penn State University Press, 2000.

Beste, Jennifer Erin. *God and the Victim: Traumatic Intrusions on Grace and Freedom (AAR Academy Series).* Oxford: Oxford University Press, 2007.

Bettenhausen, Elizabeth. "Hagar Revisited: Surrogacy, Alienation, and Motherhood." *Christianity and Crisis* 47 (May 1987): 157–59.

Blyth, Eric. "'I Wanted to Be Interesting. I Wanted to Be Able to Say "I've Done Something Interesting with My Life"': Interviews with Surrogate Mothers in Britain." *Journal of Reproductive and Infant Psychology* 12 (1994): 189–98.

Board for Social Responsibility. *Human Fertilization and Embryology: The Response of the Board for Social Responsibility of the General Synod of the Church of England to the DHSS Report of the Committee of Inquiry.* London: Board for Social Responsibility, 1984.

Booty, John J., and Stephen Sykes. *The Study of Anglicanism.* Rev. ed. Minneapolis: Fortress/SPCK, 1998.

Bracken, Joseph A. *The Triune Symbol: Persons, Process, and Community.* Lanham, Md.: University Press of America, 1985.

Brison, Susan J. *Aftermath: Violence and the Remaking of a Self.* Princeton: Princeton University Press, 2003.

———. "Personal Identity and Relational Selves." In *The Routledge Companion to Feminist Philosophy*, edited by Ann Garry, Serene J. Khader, and Alison Stone, 218–30. Basingstoke, U.K.: Taylor & Francis, 2017.

Bromell, David J. "Sallie McFague's 'Metaphorical Theology.'" *Journal of the American Academy of Religion* 61, no. 3 (1993): 485–503.

Browning, Don S. *A Fundamental Practical Theology: Descriptive and Strategic Proposal.* Minneapolis: Fortress, 1991.

———, ed. *Practical Theology: The Emerging Field in Theology, Church and World.* San Francisco: Harper & Row, 1983.

Browning, Don S., Bonnie Miller-McLemore, Pamela D. Couture, K. Brynolf Lyon, and Robert M. Franklin. *From Culture Wars to Common Ground: Religion and the American Family Debate.* Louisville: Westminster John Knox, 1997.

Butler, Judith. *Gender Trouble: Feminism and the Subversion of Identity.* New York: Routledge, 2015.

Cahill, Lisa Sowle. "Embodying God's Image: Created, Broken, and Redeemed." In *Humanity Before God: Contemporary Faces of Jewish, Christian, and Islamic Ethics,* edited by William Schweiker, Michael A. Johnson, and Kevin Jung. Minneapolis: Fortress, 2006.

———. *Family: A Christian Social Perspective.* Minneapolis: Fortress, 2000.

———. *Theological Bioethics: Participation, Justice, and Change.* Washington, D.C.: Georgetown University Press, 2005.

Callaway, Mary. *Sing, O Barren One.* Atlanta: Scholars Press, 1986.

Cameron, Nigel M. de S., ed. *Embryos and Ethics.* Edinburgh: Rutherford House Books, 1987.

Caplan, Arthur, Robert George. "Ethical Questions: Test Tube Babies." WGBH American Experience. July 13, 2012. http://www.pbs.org/wgbh/americanexperience/features/interview/ethical-questions/.

Carney, Scott. *The Red Market: On the Trail of the World's Organ Brokers, Bone Thieves, Blood Farmers, and Child Traffickers.* New York: William Morrow, 2011.

Carr, Anne. *Transforming Grace: Christian Tradition and Women's Experience.* San Francisco: Harper & Row, 1988.

Carter, Warren. "'The Blind, Lame, and Paralyzed' (John 5:3): John's Gospel, Disability Studies, and Postcolonial Perspectives." In *Disability Studies and Biblical Literature*, edited by Jeremy Schipper and Candida R. Moss, 129–50. New York: Palgrave Macmillan, 2011.

Caruth, Cathy, ed. *Trauma: Explorations in Memory.* Baltimore: The Johns Hopkins University Press, 1995.

———*Unclaimed Experience: Trauma, Narrative, and History.* Baltimore: The Johns Hopkins University Press, 1996.

Catholic Church. *Catechism of the Catholic Church: Revised in Accordance with the Official Latin Text Promulgated by Pope John Paul II.* Vatican City:

Libreria Editrice Vaticana, 1997. http://www.vatican.va/archive/ccc_css/archive/catechism/p3s2c2a4.htm.

Cavanaugh, William T. *Torture and Eucharist: Theology, Politics, and the Body of Christ*. Oxford: Wiley-Blackwell, 1998.

Centers for Disease Control and Prevention. "Infertility." July 15, 2016. https://www.cdc.gov/nchs/fastats/infertility.htm.

———. "National Summary and Fertility Clinic Tables." http://apps.nccd.cdc.gov/art/Apps/NationalSummaryReport.aspx. Accessed June 18, 2012.

Centers for Disease Control and Prevention, American Society for Reproductive Medicine, and Society for Assisted Reproductive Technology. *2014 Assisted Reproductive Technology National Summary Report*. Atlanta: U.S. Department of Health and Human Services, 2016.

Childress-Beatty, Lindsay. "Embryo Donation: Psychological Aspects." In Goldfarb, *Third-Party Reproduction*, 113–20.

Chopp, Rebecca S., and Sheila Greeve Davaney, eds. *Horizons in Feminist Theology Identity, Tradition, and Norms*. Minneapolis: Fortress, 2000.

Christ, Carol P., and Judith Plaskow, eds. *Womanspirit Rising: A Feminist Reader in Religion*. Chicago: HarperOne, 1992.

Church of England. *Personal Origins: The Report of a Working Party on Human Fertilisation and Embryology of the Board for Social Responsibility*. London: CIO Publishing, 1985.

Circle Surrogacy. "Anticipated Costs for Gestational Surrogacy." June 19, 2012. http://www.circlesurrogacy.com/costs.

Clark, Jawanza Eric. *Indigenous Black Theology: Toward an African-Centered Theology of the African American Religious Experience*. New York: Palgrave Macmillan, 2012.

Code, Lorraine. "Second Persons." In *What Can She Know? Feminist Theory and the Construction of Knowledge*, edited by Lorraine Code, 71–109. Ithaca, N.Y.: Cornell University Press, 1991.

Cohen, Chaim. "Studies in Extra-biblical Inscriptions I: The Semantic Range and Usage of the Terms אמה and שפחה." *Shnaton* 5–6 (1982–3): xxi–liii.

Coleman, Monica A. *Making a Way Out of No Way: A Womanist Theology*. Innovations: African American Religious Thought. Minneapolis: Fortress, 2008.

———. "Sacrifice, Surrogacy, and Salvation." *Black Theology* 12, no. 3 (2014): 200–212.

Congregation for the Doctrine of the Faith. "*Dignitas personae*: The Dignity of a Person." September 8, 2008. http://www.vatican.va/roman_curia/congregations/cfaith/documents/rc_con_cfaith_doc_20081208_dignitas-personae_en.html.

Congregation for the Doctrine of the Faith. "*Donum vitae*: Instruction on Respect for Human Life." February 22, 1987. http://www.vatican.va/roman_curia/congregations/cfaith/documents/rc_con_cfaith_doc_19870222_respect-for-human-life_en.html.

Copeland, M. Shawn. "The New Anthropological Subject at the Heart of the Mystical Body of Christ." *CTSA Proceedings* 53 (1998): 25–47.

———. "Toward a Critical Christian Feminist Theology of Solidarity." In *Women and Theology*, edited by Mary Ann Hinsdale and Phyllis H. Kaminski. Maryknoll, N.Y.: Orbis, 1995.

Corley, Stephanie O., and Jessica Wilen Berg. "Embryo Donation: Ethical Aspects." In Goldfarb, *Third-Party Reproduction*, 121–32.

Corley, Stephanie O., and Maxwell Mehlman. "Sperm Donation: Legal Aspects." In Goldfarb, *Third-Party Reproduction*, 31–40.

Craigo-Snell, Shannon, and Christopher Doucot. *No Innocent Bystander: Becoming an Ally in the Struggle for Justice.* Louisville: Westminster John Knox, 2017.

Creative Family Connections. "U.S. Surrogacy Map." http://www.creativefamilyconnections.com/us-surrogacy-law-map. Accessed October 11, 2016.

Crockin, Susan L., and Laura M. Nussbaum. "Embryo Donation: Legal Aspects." In Goldfarb, *Third-Party Reproduction*, 159–68.

Cullinan, Colleen Carpenter. *Redeeming the Story: Women, Suffering, and Christ.* New York: Continuum, 2004.

Curtiss, Susan. *Genie: A Psycholinguistic Study of a Modern-Day "Wild Child."* New York: Academic Press, 1977.

Dahl, Robert A. "The Concept of Power," *Behavioral Science* 2, no. 3 (2007): 1–15.

Daly, Martin, and Margo Wilson. *Sex, Evolution, and Behavior.* North Scituate, Mass.: Duxbury, 1978.

Derek, Julia. *Confessions of a Serial Egg Donor.* New York: Adrenaline Books, 2004.

De Vaux, Roland. *Ancient Israel: Its Life and Institutions.* Translated by John McHugh. London: Darton, Longman & Todd, 1961.

Diamond, Ronny, ed. *Couple Therapy for Infertility.* New York: Guilford Press, 1999.

Dobash, Russell P., R. Emerson Dobash, Margo Wilson, and Martin Daly. "The Myth of Sexual Symmetry in Marital Violence." *Social Problems* 39 (1992): 71–91.

Doehring, Carrie. "A Method of Feminist Pastoral Theology." In *Feminist and Womanist Pastoral Theology,* edited by Bonnie Miller-McLemore and Brita Gill-Austern, 95–112. Nashville: Abingdon, 1999.

———. *The Practice of Pastoral Care: A Postmodern Approach*. Louisville: Westminster John Knox, 2015.

Douglas, Kelly Brown. *Stand Your Ground: Black Bodies and the Justice of God*. Maryknoll, N.Y.: Orbis, 2015.

Dykstra, Craig. "Reconceiving Practice in Theological Inquiry and Education." In *Virtues and Practices in the Christian Tradition*, edited by Brad J. Kallenberg, Nancey Murphy, and Mark Thiessen Nation. Notre Dame, Ind.: University of Notre Dame Press, 1997.

Farley, Edward. *Divine Empathy: A Theology of God*. Minneapolis: Fortress, 1996.

———. *Ecclesial Reflection*. Philadelphia: Fortress, 1982.

———, ed. *Practical Theology: The Emerging Field in Theology, Church, and World*. New York: Harper & Row, 1982.

———. *Theologia: The Fragmentation of University Theological Education*. Philadelphia: Fortress, 1983.

Farley, Margaret. "New Patterns of Relationship: Beginnings of a Moral Revolution." *Theological Studies* 36, no. 4 (1975): 627–46.

Farley, Wendy. *The Wounding and Healing of Desire: Weaving Heaven and Earth*. Louisville: Westminster John Knox, 2005.

Fehr, Beverley Ann. *Friendship Processes*. Thousand Oaks, Calif.: Sage, 1999.

Fertility Treatment Abroad. "Surrogacy as an Infertility Treatment." http://fertility.treatmentabroad.com/treatments/surrogacy. Accessed October 13, 2016.

Festinger, L., S. Schachter, and K. Bach. *Social Pressures in Informal Groups*. Stanford, Calif.: Stanford University Press, 1963.

Finkelhor, David. *Sexually Victimized Children*. New York: Free Press, 1979.

Fisher, Allen. "Still 'Not Quite as Good as Having Your Own'? Toward a Sociology of Adoption." *Annual Review of Sociology* 29 (2003): 339–51.

Flynn, Michael, and Charles B. Strozier. *Trauma and Self*. Lanham, Md.: Rowman & Littlefield, 1996.

Ford, Mary. "Towards the Restoration of Allegory: Christology, Epistemology and Narrative Structure." *St. Vladimir's Theological Quarterly* 34, no. 2 (1990): 161–95.

Franco, Zeno E., Kathy Blau, and Philip G. Zimbardo. "Heroism: A Conceptual Analysis and Differentiation between Heroic Action and Altruism," *Review of General Psychology* 15, no. 2 (2011): 99–113.

Franklin, Sarah, and Helena Ragoné, eds. *Reproducing Reproduction: Kinship, Power, and Technological Innovation*. Philadelphia: University of Pennsylvania Press, 1998.

Frantz, Nadine Pence. "Why?" In Frantz and Stimming, *Hope Deferred*, 25–27.

Frantz, Nadine Pence, and Mary T. Stimming, eds. *Hope Deferred: Heart-Healing Reflections on Reproductive Loss*. Eugene, Ore.: Resource/Wipf & Stock, 2010.

Fuchs, Esther. "The Literary Characterization of Mothers and Sexual Politics in the Hebrew Bible." In *Women in the Hebrew Bible: A Reader*, edited by Alice Bach, 127–40. New York: Routledge, 1999.

Fulkerson, Mary McClintock. *Changing the Subject: Women's Discourses and Feminist Theology*. Minneapolis: Fortress, 1994.

Gafney, Wilda. *Womanist Midrash: A Reintroduction to the Women of the Torah and the Throne*. Louisville: Westminster John Knox, 2017.

GBCS Bioethics Task Force. *Spiritual Discernment: A Guide for Genetic and Reproductive Technologies*. Washington, D.C.: United Methodist Church, 2008.

Gerrity, Deborah. "A Biopsychosocial Theory of Infertility." *Family Journal* 9, no. 2 (2001): 151–58.

Gilligan, James. *Violence: Reflections on a National Epidemic*. New York: Vintage Books, 1997.

Gilling, J. *In vitro veritas*. London: St. Mary's Bourne Street, 1984.

Goldfarb, James M., ed. *Third-Party Reproduction: A Comprehensive Guide*. New York: Springer, 2013.

Graham, Elaine L. *Transforming Practice: Pastoral Theology in an Age of Uncertainty*. London: Mowbray, 1996.

Greil, Arthur L. "Infertility and Psychological Distress: A Review of the Literature." *Social Science and Medicine* 45, no. 11 (1997): 1679–704.

Greil, Arthur L., Kathleen Slauson-Blevins, and Julia McQuillan. "The Experience of Infertility: A Review of Recent Literature." *Sociology of Health & Illness* 32, no. 1 (2010): 140–62.

Griswold, Zara. *Surrogacy Was the Way: Twenty Intended Mothers Tell Their Stories*. Gurnee, Ill.: Nightengale Press, 2006.

Gugucheva, Magdalina. *Council for Responsible Genetics: Surrogacy in America*. Cambridge, Mass.: Council for Responsible Genetics, 2010.

Hackett, Jo Ann. "Can a Sexist Model Liberate Us? Ancient Near Eastern 'Fertility' Goddesses," *Journal of Feminist Studies in Religion* 5, no. 1 (1989): 65–76.

Hall, Amy Laura. *Conceiving Parenthood: American Protestantism and the Spirit of Reproduction*. Grand Rapids: Eerdmans, 2008.

Hayes, Diana L. "Standing in the Shoes My Mother Made: The Making of a Catholic Womanist Theologian." In *Deeper Shades of Purple: Womanism in Religion and Society*, edited by Stacey M. Floyd-Thompas, 54–76. New York: New York University Press, 2006.

Heimbrock, Hans-Günter. "Given through the Senses: A Phenomenological Model of Empirical Theology." In *Normativity and Empirical Research in Theology,* edited by Johannes A. van der Ven and Michael Scherer-Rath, 59–83. Leiden: Brill, 2004.

Henning, Meghan. "In Sickness and in Health: Ancient 'Rituals of Truth' in the Greco-Roman World and 1 Peter." In *Disability Studies and Biblical Literature,* edited by Jeremy Schipper and Candida R. Moss, 185–204. New York: Palgrave Macmillan, 2011.

Henslin, James M. "Craps and Magic," *American Journal of Sociology* 73, no. 3 (1967): 316–30.

Herman, Judith. *Trauma and Recovery: The Aftermath of Violence—from Domestic Abuse to Political Terror.* New York: Basic Books, 1997.

Heyward, Isabel Carter. *The Redemption of God: A Theology of Mutual Relation.* Eugene, Ore.: Wipf & Stock, 2010.

Higgins, Ilona Laszlo. *Creating Life against the Odds: The Journey from Infertility to Parenthood.* Bloomington, Ind.: Xlibris, 2006.

Hill, William J. *The Three-Personed God: The Trinity as a Mystery of Salvation.* Washington, D.C.: Catholic University of America Press, 1982.

Hirsch, Marianne. "Family Pictures: *Maus*, Mourning, and Post-memory." *Discourse* 15, no. 2 (1992–1993): 3–29.

Hofstede, Geert. "The Cultural Relativity of the Quality of Life Concept." *The Academy of Management Review* 9, no. 3 (1984): 389–98.

Hohman, Melinda M., and Christine B. Hagan. "Satisfaction with Surrogate Mothering." *Journal of Human Behavior in the Social Environment* 4 (2001): 61–84.

Hunt, Mary E. *Fierce Tenderness: A Feminist Theology of Friendship.* Minneapolis: Fortress, 2009.

Institute of Health Metrics and Evaluations. "Maternal Mortality Ratio." https://vizhub.healthdata.org/sdg/. Accessed November 4, 2017.

International Committee for Monitoring Assisted Reproductive Technology. "World Collaborative Report on Assisted Reproduction." *Human Reproduction 25, no. 5* (September 1, 2009): 2310–20. http://humrep.oxfordjournals.org/content/24/9/2310/T1.expansion.html.

Isasi-Díaz, Ada María. "Solidarity: Love of Neighbor in the 1980s." In *Lift Every Voice: Constructing Christian Theologies from the Underside,* edited by Susan B. Thistlethwaite and Mary P. Engel. San Francisco: Harper & Row, 1990.

Jacob, Sharon. *Reading Mary alongside Indian Surrogate Mothers: Violent Love, Oppressive Liberation, and Infancy Narratives.* New York: Palgrave Macmillan, 2015.

Jadva V., L. Blake, P. Casey, and S. Golombok. "Surrogacy Families 10 Years On: Relationship with the Surrogate, Decisions Over Disclosure and Children's Understanding of Their Surrogacy Origins." *Human Reproduction* 27 (2012): 3008–14.

Jadva, V., C. Murray, E. Lycett, F. MacCallum, and S. Golombok. "Surrogacy: The Experiences of Surrogate Mothers." *Human Reproduction* 18 (2003): 2196–204.

Jaffe, Janet, David Diamond, and Martha Diamond. *Unsung Lullabies: Understanding and Coping with Infertility.* New York: St. Martin's Griffin: 2005.

Jaffe, Janet, and Martha Diamond. *Reproductive Trauma: Psychotherapy with Infertility and Pregnancy Loss Clients.* Washington, D.C.: American Psychological Association, 2010.

Jarvis Thomson, Judith. "A Defense of Abortion." *Philosophy and Public Affairs* 1, no. 1 (1971): 47–66.

Johnson, Elizabeth A. *She Who Is: The Mystery of God in Feminist Theological Discourse.* 10th anniversary ed. New York: Crossroad, 2002.

Jones, Serene. "Rupture." In Frantz and Stimming, *Hope Deferred,* 47–66.

———. *Trauma and Grace: Theology in a Ruptured World.* Louisville: Westminster John Knox, 2009.

Jordan, Judith V. "The Meaning of Mutuality." In *Women's Growth in Connection: Writings from the Stone Center,* edited by Judith V. Jordan, 81–96. New York: Guilford Press, 1991.

Keller, Catherine. "Delores Williams: Survival, Surrogacy, Sisterhood, Spirit." *Union Seminary Quarterly Review* 58, nos. 3–4 (Fall 2004): 84–94.

———. *From a Broken Web: Separation, Sexism and Self.* Boston: Beacon Press, 1988.

Keshgegian, Flora A. *Redeeming Memories: A Theology of Healing and Transformation.* Nashville: Abingdon, 2000.

Khetarpal, Abha, and Satendra Singh. "Infertility: Why Can't We Classify This Inability as Disability?" *Australasian Medical Journal* 5, no. 6 (2012): 334–39.

Kittay, Eva Feder. *Love's Labor: Essays on Women, Equality, and Dependency.* New York: Routledge, 1999.

Kittrell, Dancy. "A Comparison of the Evolution of Men's and Women's Dreams in Daniel Levinson's Theory of Adult Development." *Journal of Adult Development* (1998): 105–15.

Lambert, Jean. "An 'F Factor'? The New Testament in Some White, Feminist, Christian Theological Construction." *Journal of Feminist Studies in Religion* 2 (1985): 93–113.

Lauritzen, Paul. *Pursuing Parenthood: Ethical Issues in Assisted Reproduction.* Bloomington: Indiana University Press, 1993.

Levine, Aaron D. "Self-Regulation, Compensation, and the Ethical Recruitment of Oocyte Donors." *Hastings Center Report* 40, no. 2 (2010): 25–36.

Levinson, Daniel J. *The Seasons of a Man's Life.* New York: Alfred Knopf, 1978.

———. *The Seasons of a Woman's Life.* New York: Alfred Knopf, 1996.

Lewis, Helen Block, ed. *The Role of Shame in Symptom Formation.* Hillsdale, N.J.: Psychology Press, 1987.

Linzey, Andrew. "In Defense of Diversity." In *Gays and the Future of Anglicanism: Responses to the Windsor Report,* edited by Andrew Linzey and Richard Kirker, 160–87. New York: O Books, 2005.

Livingston, Gretchen. *Childlessness Falls, Family Size Grows among Highly Educated Women.* Washington, D.C.: Pew Research Center, 2015. http://www.pewsocialtrends.org/2015/05/07/family-size-among-mothers/.

Luther, Martin. "Comfort for Women Who Have Had a Miscarriage." Translated by James Raun. In Frantz and Stimming, *Hope Deferred*, 67–70.

MacCallum, Fiona. "Embryo Donation Parents' Attitudes towards Donors: Comparison with Adoption." *Human Reproduction* 24, no. 3 (2009): 517–23.

MacCormac, Earl R. *Metaphor and Myth in Science and Religion.* Durham, N.C.: Duke University Press, 1976.

Madsen, Barbara A. *Andersen V. King Opinion.* July 26, 2006. https://www.courts.wa.gov/newsinfo/content/pdf/759341opn.pdf. Accessed October 30, 2018.

Mahlstedt, P. P. "Psychological Issues of Infertility and Assisted Reproduction." *The Urologic Clinics of North America* (1994): 557–66.

Mahmood, Saba. *Politics of Piety: The Islamic Revival and the Feminist Subject.* Princeton, N.J.: Princeton University Press, 2012.

Malm, H. M. "Paid Surrogacy: Arguments and Responses," *Public Affairs Quarterly* 3 (1989): 57–66.

Mandela, Nelson. *Long Walk to Freedom: The Autobiography of Nelson Mandela.* Boston: Little, Brown, 1994.

Manterfield, Lisa. *I'm Taking My Eggs and Going Home: How One Woman Dared to Say No to Motherhood.* Hermosa Beach, Calif.: Steel Rose Press, 2011.

March of Dimes. "Loss and Grief." http://www.marchofdimes.com/baby/loss_stillbirth.html. Accessed December 23, 2011.

Markens, Susan. *Surrogate Motherhood and the Politics of Reproduction.* Berkeley: University of California Press, 2007.

Markus, Hazel, and Paula Nurius. "Possible Selves." *American Psychologist* 41 (1986): 954–69.

Martin, Lauren Jade. *Reproductive Tourism in the United States: Creating Family in the Mother Country.* New York: Routledge, 2015.

Maslow, Abraham. *The Hierarchy of Needs.* Corby, U.K.: Institute of Management Foundation, 1998.

Maurice, Frederick Dennison. *To Build Christ's Kingdom: F. D. Maurice and His Writings.* London: Canterbury Press Norwich, 2007.

Mazor, Miriam. "Emotional Reactions to Infertility." In *Infertility: Medical, Emotional, and Social Considerations*, edited by Miriam D. Mazor and Harriet F. Simons, 23–35. New York: Human Sciences Press, 1984.

McFague, Sallie. *The Body of God: An Ecological Theology.* Minneapolis: Fortress, 1993.

———. *Metaphorical Theology: Models of God in Religious Language.* Philadelphia: Fortress, 1982.

———. *Models of God: Theology for an Ecological, Nuclear Age.* Philadelphia: Fortress, 1987.

McFarlane, Alexander C., and Bessel A. van der Kolk. "Trauma and Its Challenge to Society." In *Traumatic Stress: The Effects of Overwhelming Experience on Mind, Body, and Society*, edited by Bessel A. van der Kolk, Alexander C. McFarlane, and Lars Weisaeth, 24–46. New York: Guilford Press, 1996.

McGowan, Michelle L., and Leah Wilson. "Oocyte Donation: Ethical Aspects." In Goldfarb, *Third-Party Reproduction*, 51–60.

McGrath, Alister E. *Historical Theology: An Introduction to the History of Christian Thought.* Oxford: Wiley-Blackwell, 1998.

Meyers, Diana T, ed. *Feminists Rethink the Self.* Boulder, Colo.: Westview, 1997.

Michno, Dennis G. *A Priest's Handbook: The Ceremonies of the Church.* 3rd ed. Harrisburg, Pa.: Morehouse Publishing, 1998.

Miller, Juliet, and Jane Haynes, eds. *Inconceivable Conceptions: Psychological Aspects of Infertility and Reproductive Technology.* New York: Routledge, 2003.

Miller-McLemore, Bonnie. *Also a Mother: Work and Family as Theological Dilemma.* Nashville: Abingdon, 1994.

———. "The 'Clerical Paradigm': A Fallacy of Misplaced Concreteness?" *International Journal of Practical Theology* 11, no. 2 (2007): 19–38.

———. "Pastoral Theology and Public Theology." In *Pathways to the Public Square: Practical Theology in an Age of Pluralism*, edited by Elaine Graham and Anna Rowlands, 95–106. International Academy of Practical Theology, Manchester 2003. Münster, Ger.: LIT Verlag, 2005.

Modell, Judith. "In Search: The Purposed Biological Basis of Parenthood." *American Ethnologist* 13, no. 4 (1986): 646–61.

Moltmann-Wendell, Elisabeth. "Motherhood or Friendship." In *The Power of Naming: A Concilium Reader in Feminist Liberation Theology*, edited by Elisabeth Schüssler Fiorenza, 292–99. London: SCM Press, 1996.

Moore, James M. "What Is the Sense of Agency and Why Does It Matter?" *Frontiers in Psychology* 7 (2016): 1272.

Moore, Mary Elizabeth. "Feminist Practical Theology and the Future of the Church." In *Practical Theology: International Perspectives*, edited by Friedrich Schweitzer and J. A. van der Ven, 189–209. Frankfurt am Main: Peter Lang, 1999.

Moss, Candida R., and Joel S. Baden. *Reconceiving Infertility: Biblical Perspectives on Procreation and Childlessness*. Princeton, N.J.: Princeton University Press, 2015.

National Organ Transplant Act. Public Law 98-507. Introduced by Sen. Orrin Hatch, passed October 19, 1984. Accessed via National Institutes of Health. https://history.nih.gov/research/downloads/PL98-507.pdf.

Nelson, Derek R. *What's Wrong with Sin: Sin in Individual and Social Perspective from Schleiermacher to Theologies of Liberation*. New York: T&T Clark, 2009.

Newman, David. *Families: A Sociology Perspective*. New York: McGraw-Hill Higher Education, 2009.

Nieman, James. "Attending Locally: Theologies in Congregations." *International Journal of Practical Theology* 6, no. 2 (2002): 198–225.

O'Donovan, Oliver. *Begotten or Made?* Oxford: Clarendon, 1984.

Orenstein, Peggy. *Waiting for Daisy: A Tale of Two Continents, Three Religions, Five Infertility Doctors, an Oscar, an Atomic Bomb, a Romantic Night, and One Woman's Quest to Become a Mother*. New York: Bloomsbury, 2007.

Pagels, Elaine. "What Became of God the Mother? Conflicting Images of God in Early Christianity." In *Womanspirit Rising: A Feminist Reader in Religion*, edited by Carol Christ and Judith Plaskow, 107–20. New York: Harper & Row, 1979.

Pande, Amrita. *Wombs in Labor: Transnational Commercial Surrogacy in India*. New York: Columbia University Press, 2014.

Parker, Philip. "Motivations of Surrogate Mothers: Initial Findings," *American Journal of Psychiatry and Law* 140 (1983): 117–18.

Parks, Jennifer A. "Care Ethics and the Global Practice of Commercial Surrogacy." *Bioethics* 24, no. 7 (2010): 333–40.

Pepper, Stephen C. *World Hypotheses: A Study in Relevance*. Berkeley: University of California Press, 1961.

Peters, Ted. "McFague's Metaphors." *Dialog* 27, no. 2 (1988): 131–42.

Petok, William D. "Sperm Donation: Psychological Aspects." In Goldfarb, *Third-Party Reproduction*, 159–68.

Pitkin, Hanna F. *Wittgenstein and Justice: On the Significance of Ludwig Wittgenstein for Social and Political Thought*. Berkeley: University of Berkeley Press, 1993.

Poling, James N., and Donald Miller. *Foundations for a Practical Theology of Ministry*. Nashville: Abingdon, 1985.

Potts, Phoebe. *Good Eggs: A Memoir*. New York: Harper, 2010.

Powell, Brian, Catherine Bolzendahl, Claudia Geist, and Lala Carr Steelman. *Counted Out: Same-Sex Relations and Americans' Definitions of Family*. New York: Russell Sage Foundation, 2010.

Preciado, P., T. Snijders, W. J. Burk, H. Stattin, and M. Kerr. "Does Proximity Matter? Distance Dependence of Adolescent Friendships." *Social Networks* 34 (2011): 18–31.

Prichard, Robert. *A History of the Episcopal Church*. Rev. ed. Harrisburg, Pa.: Morehouse Publishing, 1999.

Quaas, Alexander, and Anuja Dokras, "Diagnosis and Treatment of Unexplained Infertility." *Reviews in Obstetrics and Gynecology* 1, no. 2 (Spring 2008): 69–76.

Ragoné, Helena. *Surrogate Motherhood: Conception in the Heart*. Boulder, Colo.: Westview, 1994.

Ragoné, Helena, and France Winddance Twine, eds. *Ideologies and Technologies of Motherhood: Race, Class, Sexuality, Nationalism*. New York: Routledge, 2000.

Rambo, Shelly. *Spirit and Trauma: A Theology of Remaining*. Louisville: Westminster John Knox, 2010.

———. *Resurrecting Wounds: Living in the Aftermath of Trauma*. Waco: Baylor University Press, 2017.

Ramsey, Michael. *The Gospel and the Catholic Church*. London: Longmans, Green and Co., 1936.

Raymond, Janice. *A Passion for Friends: Toward a Philosophy of Female Affection*. Boston: Beacon, 1986.

Reame N. E., A. Kalfoglou , and H. A. Hanafin. "Long Term Outcomes of Surrogate Pregnancy: A Report of Surrogate Mother's Satisfaction, Life Events and Moral Judgements Ten Years Later." *Fertility and Sterility* 70 (1998): 28–29.

RESOLVE: The National Infertility Association. "Infertility Coverage by State." RESOLVE: The National Infertility Association. http://www.resolve.org/family-building-options/insurance_coverage/infertility-coverage-state. Accessed October 30, 2018.

Reynolds, Terrence. "Parting Company at Last: Lindbeck and McFague in Substantive Theological Dialogue." *Concordia Theological Quarterly* 63, no. 2 (1999): 97–118.

Riesener, Ingrid. *Der Stamm* צבר *im Alten Testament: Eine Wortuntersuchunt unter Berucksichtigun neuerer sprachwissenschaftlicher Methoden*. Beihefte zur Zeitschrift für die Alttestamentliche Wissenschaft 149. Berlin: de Gruyter, 1979.

Robb, Christina. *This Changes Everything: The Relational Evolution in Psychology*. New York: Farrar, Strauss, and Giroux, 2006.

Roberts, Priscilla, and Peter M. Newton. "Levinsonian Studies of Women's Adult Development." *Psychology and Aging* 2, no. 2 (1987): 154–63.

Robertson, John A. *Children of Choice: Freedom and the New Reproductive Technologies*. Princeton, N.J.: Princeton University Press, 1994.

Rogers, Annie G. *The Unsayable: The Hidden Language of Trauma*. New York: Ballantine Books, 2007.

Root, Maria. "Reconstructing the Impact of Trauma on Personality." In *Personality and Psychopathology: Feminist Reappraisals*, edited by Laura S. Brown, 229–65. New York: Guilford Press, 1994.

Rosenblatt, Naomi Harris. *After the Apple: Women in the Bible—Timeless Stories of Love, Lust, and Longing*. New York: Miramax Books, 2005.

Rothman, Barbara Katz. *Recreating Motherhood*. New Brunswick, N.J.: Rutgers University Press, 2000.

Rothschild, Babette. *The Body Remembers: The Psychophysiology of Trauma and Trauma Treatment*. New York: W. W. Norton, 2000.

Rudrappa, Sharmila. "India's Reproductive Assembly Line." *Contexts* 11, no.2 (2012): 22–27.

Ruether, Rosemary Radford. *Christianity and the Making of the Modern Family*. Boston: Beacon Press, 2000.

Russell, Letty M. *Church in the Round: Feminist Interpretation of the Church*. Louisville: Westminster John Knox, 1993.

Ryan, Maura A. *Ethics and Economics of Assisted Reproduction: The Cost of Longing*. Moral Traditions Series. Washington, D.C.: Georgetown University Press, 2003.

Sachs, William L. *The Transformation of Anglicanism: From State Church to Global Communion*. Cambridge: Cambridge University Press, 2002.

Savage, Carolyn, and Sean Savage. *Inconceivable: A Medical Mistake, the Baby We Couldn't Keep, and Our Choice to Deliver the Ultimate Gift*. New York: HarperOne, 2011.

Schwartz, Baruch J. The *Holiness Legislation: Studies in the Priestly Code*. Jerusalem: Magnes, 1999.

———. "A Literary Study of the Slave-Girl Pericope—Leviticus 19:20-22." In *Studies in the Bible 1986, Scripta Hierosolymitana* 31, edited by Sara Japhet, 241–55. Jerusalem: Magnes, 1986.

Schweitzer, Friedrich. "Practical Theology, Contemporary Culture, and the Social Sciences: Interdisciplinary Relationships and the Unity of Practical Theology as a Discipline." In *Normativity and Empirical Research in Theology*, edited by Johannes A. van der Ven and Michael Scherer-Rath, 307–21. Leiden: Brill, 2004.

Sclater, Shelley Day. *Surrogate Motherhood: International Perspectives*. Edited by Rachel Cook. Portland, Ore.: Hart Publishing, 2003.

Scott, Ken, dir. *Delivery Man*. Film. New York: DreamWorks, 2013.

Shalev, Carmel. "An Ethic of Care and Responsibility: Reflections on Third-Party Reproduction." *Medicine Studies* 3, no. 3 (2012): 147–56.

Sharma, Rahul. "The Family and Family Structure Classification Redefined for the Current Times." *Journal of Family Medicine and Primary Care* 2, no. 4 (2013): 306–10.

Siegel, Daniel J. *The Developing Mind: How Relationships and the Brain Interact to Shape Who We Are*. 2nd ed. New York: Guilford Press, 2012.

Simmel, Georg. *The Philosophy of Money*. London: Routledge and Keagan Paul, 1978.

Smith, Andrea. *Conquest: Sexual Violence and American Genocide*. Durham: Duke University Press, 2015.

Smith, Daniel Scott. "Family Limitation, Sexual Control, and Domestic Feminism in Victorian America." In *Controlling Reproduction: An American History*, edited by Andrea Tone, 77–98. Lanham, Md.: Rowman & Littlefield, 1996.

Smith, David H., ed. *Caring Well: Religion, Narrative, and Health Care Ethics*. Louisville: Westminster John Knox, 2000.

———. *Health and Medicine in the Anglican Tradition*. New York: Crossroad, 1986.

———. "Medical Loyalty: Dimensions and Problems of a Rich Idea." In *Theology and Bioethics: Exploring the Foundations and* Frontiers, edited by E. E. Shelp, 267–82. Boston: D. Reidel, 1985.

———. *Partnership with the Dying: Where Medicine and Ministry Should Meet*. Lanham, Md.: Rowman & Littlefield, 2005.

———. *Religious Giving: For Love of God*. Bloomington: Indiana University Press, 2010.

Sokoloff, Burton Z. "Antecedents of American Adoption." *The Future of Children* 3, no. 1 (1993): 17–25. doi:10.2307/1602399.

Spar, Debora L. *The Baby Business: How Money, Science, and Politics Drive the Commerce of Conception*. Boston: Harvard Business Review Press, 2006.

Standing Commission on Liturgy and Music. *Liturgies and Prayers Related to Childbearing, Childbirth, and Loss: Enriching Our Worship 5*. New York: Church, 2010.

Starr, Lee Anna. *The Bible Status of Woman*. New York: Fleming H. Revell, 1926.

Stewart, Dianne M. "Womanist God-Talk on the Cutting Edge of Theology and Black Religious Studies Assessing the Contribution of Delores Williams." *Union Seminary Quarterly Review* 58, nos. 3–4 (Fall 2004): 65–83.

Stimming, Mary T. "Sorrow." In Frantz and Stimming, *Hope Deferred*, 33–35.

Stone, Bryan P. *Evangelism after Christendom: The Theology and Practice of Christian Witness*. Maryknoll, N.Y.: Orbis, 2007.

Stringer, Martin. "The Many Faces of Anglicanism." In *Gays and the Future of Anglicanism: Responses to the Windsor Report*, edited by Andrew Linzey and Richard Kirker. New York: O Books, John Hunt, 2005.

Stuckey, Johanna H. "Ancient Mother Goddesses and Fertility Cults," *Journal of the Association for Research on Mothering* 7, no. 1 (2005): 32–44.

Stuhlman, Byron David. *Occasions of Grace: An Historical and Theological Study of the Pastoral Offices and Episcopal Services in the Book of Common Prayer*. New York: Church Publishing, 1995.

Suchoki, Marjorie Hewitt. *The Fall to Violence*. New York: Continuum, 1995.

———. "Openness and Mutuality in Process Thought and Feminist Action." In *Feminist and Process Thought*, edited by Sheila G. Davaney. New York: Edwin Mellen, 1981.

Surrey, Janet L. "The 'Self-in-Relation': A Theory of Women's Development." In *Women's Growth in Connection: Writings from the Stone Center*, edited by Judith V. Jordan. New York: Guilford Press, 1991.

"Surrogate Mother Compensation." Surrogacy America. https://www.surrogacyamerica.com/become-surrogate-mother/surrogate-mother-compensation. Accessed March 03, 2017.

"Surrogate Mother Pay: Compensation for Surrogate Mothers." Conceive-Abilities. https://www.conceiveabilities.com/surrogates/ surrogate-mother-pay. Accessed March 03, 2017.

Swinton, John. *Becoming Friends of Time: Disability, Timefullness, and Gentle Discipleship*. Waco, Tex.: Baylor University Press, 2017.

———. *Raging with Compassion: Pastoral Responses to the Problem of Evil*. London: SCM Press, 2018.

Swinton, John, and Harriet Mowat. *Practical Theology and Qualitative Research*. London: SCM Press, 2006.

Tal, Kalí. *Worlds of Hurt: Reading the Literatures of Trauma*. Cambridge Studies in American Literature and Culture. Cambridge: Cambridge University Press, 1995.

Teman, Elly. *Birthing a Mother: The Surrogate Body and the Pregnant Self.* Berkeley: University of California Press, 2010.

Terrell, JoAnne Marie. *Power in the Blood? The Cross in the African American Experience*. Eugene, Ore.: Wipf & Stock, 2005.

TeSelle, Sallie McFague. *Speaking in Parables: A Study in Metaphor and Theology*. Philadelphia: Fortress, 1975.

Traina, Cristina L. H. *Feminist Ethics and Natural Law: The End of the Anathemas*. Washington, D.C.: Georgetown University Press, 1999.

Trible, Phyllis. *Texts of Terror: Literary-Feminist Readings of Biblical Narratives*. Philadelphia: Fortress, 1984.

Turner, Amanda J., and Adrian Coyle. "What Does It Mean to Be a Donor Offspring? The Identity Experiences of Adults Conceived by Donor Insemination and the Implications for Counseling and Therapy." *Human Reproduction* 15, no. 9 (2000): 2041–51.

United States Census Bureau. "Figure FM-3: Average Number of Children per Family." In Families and Living Arrangements. https://www.census.gov/content/dam/Census/library/visualizations/time-series/demo/families-and-households/fm-3.pdf.

United States Conference of Catholic Bishops. "Instruction *Dignitas personae* on Certain Bioethical Questions." December 12, 2008. www.usccb.org/comm/Dignitaspersonae/Dignitas_Personae.pdf.

United States Department of Health and Human Services. "Family Reunification: What the Evidence Shows." *Child Welfare Information Gateway: Issues*. 2011. https://www.quantumunitsed.com/get-material.php?id=444. Accessed October 30, 2018.

United States Equal Employment Opportunity Commission. "The Pregnancy Discrimination Act of 1978." Approved October 31, 1978. https://www.eeoc.gov/laws/statutes/pregnancy.cfm.

van der Kolk, Bessel A. "The Body Keeps the Score: Memory and the Emerging Psychobiology of Post-traumatic Stress." *Harvard Review of Psychiatry* 1, no. 5 (January–February 1994): 253–65.

van der Kolk, Bessel, Alexander C. McFarlane, and Lars Weisaeth, eds. *Traumatic Stress: The Effects of Overwhelming Experience on Mind, Body, and Society*. New York: Guilford Press, 2007.

van der Ven, Johannes A. "An Empirical or a Normative Approach to Practical-Theological Research? A False Dilemma." In *Normativity and Empirical Research in Theology,* edited by Johannes A. van der Ven and Michael Scherer-Rath, 101–35. Leiden: Brill, 2004).

———*Practical Theology: An Empirical Approach.* Kampen, Neth.: Kok Pharos, 1990.

———. "An Empirical Approach in Practical Theology." In *Practical Theology: International Perspectives*, edited by Friedrich Schweitzer and J. A. van der Ven, 323–39. Frankfurt am Main: Peter Lang, 2004.

van Regenmorter, John, and Sylvia Van Regenmorter. *When the Cradle Is Empty: Coping with Infertility.* Carol Stream, Ill.: Tyndale House, 2004.

Volf, Miroslav. *The End of Memory: Remembering Rightly in a Violent World.* Grand Rapids: Eerdmans, 2006.

———. *Free of Charge: Giving and Forgiving in a Culture Stripped of Grace.* Grand Rapids: Zondervan, 2006.

Volf, Miroslav, and Dorothy C. Bass, eds. *Practicing Theology: Beliefs and Practices in Christian Life.* Grand Rapids: Eerdmans, 2002.

von Rad, Gerhard. *Genesis.* Translated by John H. Marks. Philadelphia: Westminster, 1956.

Wahba, Mahmoud A., and Lawrence G. Bridwell. "Maslow Reconsidered: A Review of Research on the Need Hierarchy Theory." *Organizational Behavior and Human Performance* 15, no. 2 (1976): 212–40.

Ward, Keith. "Ecclesial Authority and Morality." In *Gays and the Future of Anglicanism: Responses to the Windsor Report*, edited by Andrew Linzey and Richard Kirker, 17–29. New York: O Books, 2005.

———. *A History of Global Anglicanism.* New York: Cambridge University Press, 2006.

Warnock, Mary, ed. *A Question of Life: The Warnock Report on Human Fertilisation and Embryology.* Oxford, U.K.: Wiley-Blackwell, 1985.

Weaver, J. Denny. *The Nonviolent Atonement.* Grand Rapids: Eerdmans, 2001.

Weingarten, Kaethe. "Witnessing, Wonder, and Hope." *Family Process* 39, no. 4 (2004): 389–402.

Weisz, Carolyn. "Social Identities and Response to Treatment for Alcohol and Cocaine Abuse." *Addictive Behaviors* 21, no.4 (1996): 445–58.

Weisz, Carolyn, and Lisa F. Wood. "Social Identity Support and Friendship Outcomes: A Longitudinal Study Predicting Who Will Be Friends and Best Friends Four Years Later." *Journal of Personal and Social Relationships* 22, no. 3 (2005): 416–32.

Wendell, Susan. *The Rejected Body: Feminist Philosophical Reflections on Disability.* New York: Routledge, 1996.

West, Cornel. *Hope on a Tightrope: Words and Wisdom.* Carlsbad, Calif.: Hay House, 2008.

West, Traci. "When a White Man-God Is the Truth and the Way." In *Christology and Whiteness: What Would Jesus Do?* edited by George Yancy, 114–27. New York: Routledge, 2012.

Westerfield-Tucker, Karen. "When the Cradle Is Empty: Rites Acknowledging Stillbirth, Miscarriage, and Infertility." *Worship* 76 (2002): 482–502.

Westermann, Claus. *The Promise to the Fathers.* Philadelphia: Fortress, 1980.

White, Deborah Gray. *Ar'n't I a Woman? Female Slaves in the Plantation South.* New York: Norton, 1985.

White, Kayla. "The Legal Status of Barren Wives in the Ancient Near East." *Priscilla Papers* 28, no. 4 (2014): 18–22.

White, Lynn. "Stepfamilies Over the Life Course: Social Support." In *Sociology of Families: Readings*, edited by Cheryl Albers, 380–87. London: Pine Forge, 1999.

Williams, Delores S. *Sisters in the Wilderness: The Challenge of Womanist God-Talk.* Maryknoll, N.Y.: Orbis, 1995.

Winkler, Cathy. "Rape as Social Murder." *Anthropology Today* 7, no. 3 (1991): 12–14.

Wolfteich, Claire. *Navigating New Terrain: Work and Women's Spiritual Lives.* New York: Paulist Press, 2002.

Woodward, Shannon. *Inconceivable: Finding Peace in the Midst of Infertility.* Colorado Springs, Colo.: David C. Cook, 2006.

World Council of Churches. *Baptism, Eucharist, and Ministry.* Geneva: World Council of Churches, 1982.

World Health Organization (WHO), United Nations Children's Fund (UNICEF), United Nations Population Fund (UNFPA), World Bank Group, and the United Nations Population Division. *Division Trends in Maternal Mortality: 1990 to 2015. Estimates by the WHO, UNICEF, UNFPA, World Bank Group and the United Nations Population Division.* http://apps.who.int/iris/bitstream/10665/194254/1/9789241565141_eng.pdf.

Yoo, Philip Y. "Hagar the Egyptian: Wife, Handmaid, and Concubine." *Catholic Biblical Quarterly* 78 (2016): 215–35.

Young, Pamela Dickey. *Re-Creating the Church: Communities of Eros.* Harrisburg, Pa.: Trinity Press International, 2000.

Zelizer, Vivian. *Pricing the Priceless Child.* New York: Basic Books, 1985.

Zizioulas, John D. *Being as Communion: Studies in Personhood and the Church.* Crestwood, N.Y.: St. Vladimir's Seminary Press, 1997.

Index